ENDORSEMENTS

"Confronting cancer unleashes a storm of emotions, fears, and stress. Confusion, anger, and a sense of aloneness and isolation are the norm. In *Cancer: What To Do Or Say*, Claudia Mulcahy shares her journey through these challenges. What she learned and shares will empower anyone who finds themselves in a similar situation. This book is crammed with terrific advice, served up with grit, humor, and a light heart. Learn from it!"

Larry Dossey, MD
Executive Editor: *Explore: The Journal of Science and Healing*
Author of *One Mind*

"A testament to how each person's experience with cancer is their own, yet often has common overlapping themes with experiences of others with cancer or other challenges in life. Claudia's story highlights how emotional support can come from numerous, and sometimes unexpected, sources, including the chance to just tell the story."

Scott A. Irwin, MD, PhD; FAPM; FAPA
Director, Psychiatry & Psychosocial Services; Patient & Family Support Services, UC San Diego Moores Cancer Center
Director, Palliative Care Psychiatry, UC San Diego Health System
Associate Professor of Clinical Psychiatry,
UC San Diego School of Medicine

"Enduring the seemingly endless struggle of battling cancer can be a mind-numbing experience for anyone afflicted with the disease. The uplifting book by Claudia Mulcahy provides a mesmerizing insight into one woman's journey with an ample spread of humor, suspense, and always a will to enlighten the reader. Both patient and caregiver will learn something and find inspiration to push them through the trials of their treatment. In addition, those with any other kinds of hardships will also have something to gain from reading this book."

Alexander V. Prokhorov, MD, PhD and
Ina N. Prokhorov, MD
The University of Texas MD Anderson Cancer Center

"Claudia's telling of her cancer saga is insightful, funny, heart-breaking, and amazing. This captivating story is peppered with clear advice for cancer patients and their caregivers. These bullets of advice are at the same time very specific to cancer but also universal. No matter how much you know about cancer, there is something to learn here."

Richard Schwab, MD
Division of Hematology/Oncology
Associate Clinical Professor of Medicine
UC San Diego Moores Cancer Center

"Those who live the experience know the territory and can be our guides, and coach us through life's trouble spots. The benefits apply to more than just cancer--so read, learn, and survive."

Bernie Siegel, MD
Author of *Love, Medicine and Miracles* and
The Art of Healing

"Claudia, you shared very well who and how you let loved ones in on your situation. I believe your thought process and it's written delivery is informative, sensitive, and well delivered (realistic). For me it is helpful for those who have yet to walk this path. It shows that courage comes in many forms. I like it."
Raymond S. Brown Sr.
Family member and friend of four who passed away from cancer

"Claudia hits the mark right on! Her book explains it clearly and made it fun to read without blowing off how frightening cancer is. This book has to get out there! Claudia walks on down the path of chemotherapy, brightening the dark spots with flashes of humor, showing us there is light at the end of the tunnel. Very well done."
Doris Enright
Patient with lung cancer

"Having lost my mother-in-law to cancer, I was excited to see Claudia share her insights into how family and friends need to interact with the patient. People don't know whether or not to talk about the illness and how to act around the patient, so they stay away. Come close, offer support, bring meals, sing songs, keep life as close to what it used to be as possible."
Jan Garrison, RN

"I recommend this book to anyone who is seeking honest, practical, useful information in dealing with a diagnosis of cancer. Claudia invites the reader to journey with her through her personal experiences, and offers insight into issues, which are rarely addressed in other books. By weaving humor throughout, Claudia encourages the reader to take a breath, to smile."
Peg Selover
Animal Reiki Practitioner and Legal Assistant

CANCER:

What to Do or Say

Claudia Mulcahy

Cancer:
What to Do or Say

Copyright © 2015 by Claudia Mulcahy

All rights reserved. No part of this book may be used or reproduced by any means, graphic, electronic, or mechanical, including photocopying, recording, taping, or by any information storage retrieval system without the written permission of the publisher except in the case of brief quotations embodied in critical articles and reviews.

ISBN: 978-0-9822331-8-4
ISBN: 0982233183
Library of Congress Control Number: 2015935934

The information, ideas, and suggestions in this book are not intended as a substitute for professional advice. Before following any suggestions contained in this book, consult your physician or mental health professional. Neither the author nor the publisher shall be liable or responsible for any loss or damage allegedly arising as a consequence of your use or application of any information or suggestions in this book.

Cover and text design: Jeaneen Lund and Miko Radcliffe
Inside photos provided by: Claudia Mulcahy
Back cover photo: Sandy Radom

Sacred Life Publishers™
SacredLife.com
Printed in the United States of America

*With gratitude,
to my parents, my Spirit Guides,
and to you, the reader.*

*And to Christine and Mary.
Thank you for being on my path in life.
You made a difference.
Peace.*

CONTENTS

Endorsements

Dedication vii

Introduction xi

With Gratitude xiii

Chapter 1 Cancer—And Other Words People Avoid 1

Chapter 2 April Fool's 11

Chapter 3 From Optimist to Ostrich 19

Chapter 4 An Appointment with Charlie Brown's Teacher 23

Chapter 5 Remorse in the Frozen Food Aisle 27

Chapter 6 Stocking Up on Toilet Paper 37

Chapter 7 A Port in the Storm 51

Chapter 8 How Spirit Showed Up For Me 63

Chapter 9 God Throws a Party 69

Chapter 10 Ch-Ch-Ch-Chai! 85

Chapter 11 Field Trip! 101

Chapter 12 Eggs, Please 113

Chapter 13 Little Victories 123

Chapter 14 Disappointments 131

Chapter 15 The Couch 139

Chapter 16 Other Great Friends 149

Chapter 17 Emerging From the Fog 165

Chapter 18 Chin Over the Bar 169

Chapter 19 Email Celebrations	175
Chapter 20 Now What?	183
Chapter 21 Where's Gallagher?	189
Chapter 22 My Mastectomy – Take Two	195
Chapter 23 After the Earthquake	213
Chapter 24 Rebuilding Barbie	221
Chapter 25 Lymphedema: Just the Facts, Ma'am	229
Chapter 26 Man Made; Never "Fake" – A Year Later	235
Chapter 27 Tassel Twirling Lessons Postponed	257
Chapter 28 I Know There's a Pony in This Pile!	261
Epilogue	263
Resources	273
About the Author	277

INTRODUCTION

This book is written for any newly diagnosed cancer patient, and for those who love them. The majority of tips in this book are appropriate for all types of cancer, with some being more specific to female breast cancer (which was my personal experience). I have since had friends diagnosed with other types of cancer, and the tips in this book worked well for them. I hope you benefit from this book.

On April 7, (two days after Palm Sunday) I was diagnosed with Stage 3 breast cancer. I was a minister, and while I lean towards mystic, and metaphysical, I felt very in tune with the Easter story, especially Maundy Thursday when Jesus prays, "If this cup cannot pass, and if I must drink it, let it be according to thy will." Matthew 26:39-42. Then, Good Friday: Sometimes rotten stuff happens to good people. Sometimes they see it coming and can do nothing about it, but hope it's part of their higher purpose. Still, that doesn't stop the fear. I knew death via this experience wasn't my purpose. I told the doctors time and again it wasn't death I feared; it was the process of treatment, and fear of mutilation. Then came my personal Easter message: Good can come out of anything. I can rise above this. There will be celebration and newness.

When diagnosed, I searched for books on cancer. Thousands of books have been written. I didn't buy one of them. I found them too medical, holistic, frilly, angry, or written from the standpoint of a martyr. I hated the textbook drawings, and the fear based stories of the "dangerous" western medical model from hard-core naturopath authors. I couldn't relate to the very feminine books oozing with estrogen, or the women venting in rage at their bodies. There wasn't a book out there for me. I had no idea what to do, or what to tell people who asked me, "How may I help you?"

They say, "Cancer changes everything." They aren't joking. My intention is to walk you through the cancer experience, while providing tips for your creating as much ease and grace as possible. Some seem to cope with cancer by laughing it off. Some are able to work, go places and continue with a social calendar. Others seem to cry or sleep their way through it, pulling out of all social circles. Not much information is written about people who don't laugh their way to health, or get back on the bike just out of chemo. Some of us crawl to the finish line. Even crawling can be done with some amount of grace.

No two people will experience this journey the same way. If this book resonates with you, please share it with others during treatments, support groups, in the waiting room, and with family, friends, neighbors, and co-workers.

I wish you peace. Deep Peace.
I wish you health, and happiness.
Blessings to you, and to those who help you.

Claudia

WITH GRATITUDE

Many thanks to all on my gratitude list, (which became my "Wall of Gratitude" covering a living room wall). You were very much a part of my healing process. Your inspiration and enthusiasm made this book a reality.

I am extremely blessed to have the relationship I do with my parents. For your love, respect, humor and my upbringing, I give thanks.

Thank you Christine, for shining your light; for leading the way. I watched you. You showed me the ropes—even your wigs, and reconstruction—and it lessened my fear. Your pixie hair growing back gave me hope in a timeline. Your visiting me on my first day of chemo gave me strength. You were a lovely lady.

My medical team gets gold stars. Thank you for consistently being awake and aware, not just professionally, but as individuals.

Synchronicity (breadcrumb-blessings) led me to the right people at the right time. Thanks to C.L. Woodhams and Writer's Bloc for inviting me to the critique group—and inviting me back. Thanks to Cheryl Brown, small business developer for helping me set up social media and keeping me on track to get the book published. You have the perfect mix of empathy and push. Thank you editor Jessica Greene, and the Sacred Life Publishers team—specifically Sharon Lund, Jeaneen Lund, and Miko Radcliffe. What a delight to work with you! I appreciate your abilities, integrity, enthusiasm and heart-centeredness.

Sandy Radom, thank you for taking my headshot, and for granting me my requests of early morning, outside, and a quick photo shoot. For this and your friendship I am blessed.

Thank you, Doctors Larry Dossey, Scott Irwin, Alexander and Ina Prokhorov, Richard Schwab, and Bernie Siegel for your support and endorsements. It's an honor. Through lending your name and comments to my work, many will pick up this book. Thanks also to Raymond S. Brown, Sr., Doris Enright, Jan Garrison, and Peg Selover. You've walked this path personally or with a loved one. Your endorsements relating to your experiences will help others looking for a book to which they can relate.

To friends and family who generously gave their time reading various drafts of this book, and offering points of clarity. Thank you.

To caregivers reading this: Thank you for taking action; for moving from feeling awkward into being of service. To patients: Thumbs up! You help pave the path for future patients. Know you're loved, and that the experience called cancer affects many more than the individual diagnosed. To all involved: Thank you for caring, reading and sharing.

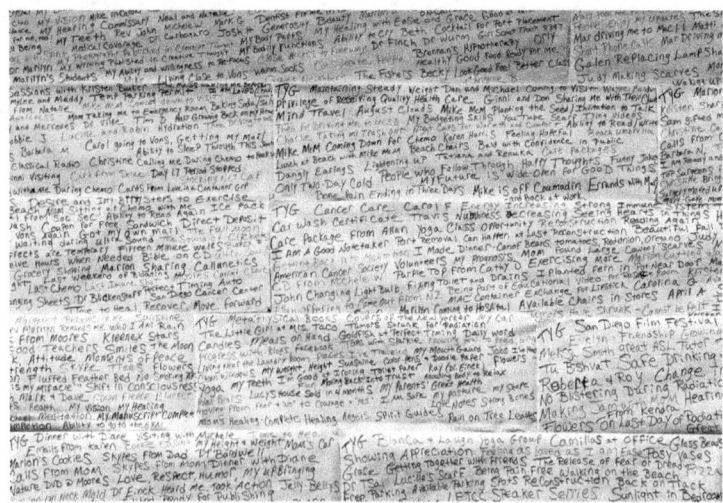

Wall of Gratitude

Chapter 1

CANCER—AND OTHER WORDS PEOPLE AVOID

"Is there any way this could be something mimicking cancer?"

The surgeon gave me her full attention. Shaking her head she said, "No."

Under my breath, I muttered, "Fuuck." And again as my head and shoulders sagged. How could this be? And again, as I saw the shock on my mother's face from the corner of my eye—the words were sinking in.

Neither resident nor surgeon flinched. I wonder if the resident thumbed through the intake form to review the answer I gave to his question, "Occupation?"

"Minister."

"I won't do chemo. I'll go to Africa and die with the elephants." The surgeon must be used to this type of response. She sat patiently as if counting to ten, waiting for my return. Somewhere between her voice and that of Charlie Brown's teacher (Whaa-whaa-whaa) I heard, Stage 3. With recommended treatment prognosis is very good. The idea of skipping treatment and going to Africa stayed in my mind as an option, but now I was able to listen and take notes.

After almost a year of noticing bumps grow and multiply in my underarm, I'd spent the past month seeing doctors over here; specialists over there. When intake nurses, or doctors asked me of family cancer history, I responded, "None." They weren't going to have what I saw as an "easy out" for a diagnosis. I didn't see it as a lie. I saw it as protection from misdiagnosis.

Because I didn't believe or trust the first one, there I was sitting in front of a surgeon for a second opinion. This was the first appointment I brought someone with me (my mom). A resident doctor came in and asked some background questions before informing the surgeon, then returning to the room with her.

One of the questions, "Anyone in the family ever been diagnosed with breast cancer?"

I stayed quiet, waiting for the shoe to drop. Mom answered, "I have." The urge to lean away, cock my head, and look incredulous crossed my mind . . . .

There. It was done. Cat out of the bag. They were serious about this cancer stuff.

Ten years earlier, my mom had a tumor in her breast 0.5 millimeter in size. She had a lumpectomy and radiation for the stage of cancer called "in situ" (a tumor that hasn't spread beyond where it originally developed). She was extremely private about her cancer, partly due to being an elected college board member at an increasingly tense time, and partly, due to the times of our society. At the time, no one was running around with pink or yellow plastic bracelets—let alone allowing the media to hear the word "cancer" during an election year. Five days after my mom had the lumpectomy, she was at a black-tie awards dinner, with drains pinned to her bra straps—no one asked how she was, or showed her extra care. No one knew. I was living in New Zealand, and had no idea what any of this meant, and again, she didn't share much. That's just how our family rolls.

The surgeon walked me though some of what the first doctor had, but pausing between levels of information for me to absorb as much as possible; showing me a 4.5-centimeter diagram for the size of the tumor; handing me a box of Kleenex when she described a mastectomy.

Chapter 1

On the way out, I was handed a barium drink with instructions for later use before a CAT Scan, and a list of various appointments to make before a follow-up with the surgeon. My mom and I left the appointment desk. I got two steps into the hallway before my legs gave out. There were benches right there—I melted into one. Seemingly from out of nowhere, yet from the innermost depths, I gasped for air, then began sobbing convulsively. It finally hit. I had cancer. They say I'd have one breast removed. They say I'd have chemotherapy. I think what set me off was seeing the two white rocking chairs in the hallway with pink well-wishes written on them. My eyes caught: You Are Loved. You Have Courage. You Are Strong. Mom stood next to me, putting her cool hand on my fevered forehead, as I continued sobbing, not giving a shit if anyone heard (and it would be a far stretch to think they didn't). My mom returned to the waiting room to get me water. I pulled it together, then we continued down the hall to get my blood drawn and eventually to the car. We'd each taken notepads into the doctor's appointment. I had several pages of timelines, doctors' names, and unfamiliar terms. I looked over at my mom's notepad: It had the two doctors' names. My heart ached for the shock she'd just encountered.

In March 2008, I was tired and couldn't shake it. Living three miles from work, I began coming home during lunch for power-naps. For dinner I'd have cereal to minimize preparation and clean up so I could go to bed early. I started going to a holistic chiropractor for Nutrition Response Testing™, a method of analyzing the body's nutritional needs through muscle response. I paid out of pocket $1,000.00 for appointments and probably another $1,000.00 on supplements my body responded as needing.

A friend dragged me to a seminar addressing diets for body types. Apparently, I needed more protein, and specifically from beef. I'd had a low fat, near-vegetarian diet for thirty years, sometimes eating chicken or fish. Just for the record, we're supposed to have three ounces (just over eighty-five grams) of protein a meal, not a day—and I doubt I even obtained that amount. I was desperate, so I began eating beef. I followed the directions: For the first two weeks, eat three ounces of beef at each meal. Yuck. I made a special trip to a "real" butcher and explained I was freaking out about the taste, texture, and the whole idea. I left with a nine-ounce filet mignon, lasting me my first three meals. My energy did in fact go up, but it didn't last.

In June, I noticed small bumps in my armpit. I thought I had a cold, or an infection; an energy block of some sort. The bumps grew. The chiropractor muscle tested me for "breast issues." No response, meaning all was well.

In October, I took my mom to Norway for a cruise along the Norwegian coast, followed by four days on land. On the cruise, I could see and feel that the bumps had increased again in size, and a new bump had formed. The largest was about the size of a large peach-pit. The others were the size of a grape, and a pea. (Food is so good for reference, isn't it?)

Soon after returning from Norway, I left the chiropractor and began acupressure. I was advised to ice the bumps. Man, this was a stubborn energy block or infection! I had no idea that bumps were a possible sign of cancer. Cancer wasn't even on my radar.

In January and March I even saw two psychics to try to figure out what was going on with these bumps. One said if I didn't do something about them, I'd get very sick. She did Reiki. I don't even like Reiki, but I found myself getting a treatment from her—once. Nice lady, but it wasn't the avenue for me. The other psychic assured me they were cysts. Not to worry.

No one was saying the word "cancer." No lights were going on for me.

My prayer partner and I continued to pray for the cause and effect of the bumps to be removed. (The last heard from her was during my first week of chemo. She left a message saying how stressed she was about various things, signing off with, "I know all is well with you.")

Chapter 1

The reason I share all this isn't to lay blame on anyone, myself included. It's to share that I knew something needed attention, yet, I didn't have a clue of what was going on. The "C" word is still very big in our society. Not one person mentioned the word "cancer" and I probably would've blown them off if anyone had. I had no intention to go to a doctor for cryin' out loud! I was healthy and happy. I ate fruit, vegetables and exercised. I never smoked and I tend to see the glass half full, rather than half empty.

During this time I didn't have health insurance. COBRA "coverage" would've cost over $1,300 a month, and excluded any back, neck, or heart coverage due to spine surgery for scoliosis in the seventies, and an outpatient heart procedure (radiofrequency ablation - RFA) to slow a fast heartbeat in the early 2000s. When I left my job in 2007, I knew COBRA wasn't an option. In 2008, I poured my money into my start-up company. I was healthy and knew I'd eventually have coverage. There was no doubt in my mind I was fine.

In March, "out of the blue", I realized someone in the medical field needed to check out my situation. I had no idea where to go, or even the purpose of the visit. Did I go to a dermatologist? Or someone who dealt with infections (which is what I believed my case to be)? I'd gone nine months with bumps in my underarm. Then, for two mornings in a row, I had pain in my breasts when I rolled over onto my stomach in bed. (I never lie on my stomach!) The second morning, I looked to see what was causing the problem. One breast was peeling and looked just a little different.

Later that day I searched the Internet to see if I could find a local medical clinic. I'd never been to one, but figured it would be less expensive, and without health insurance, the place to start. I scheduled with the nurse practitioner, drawn to the fact she was from New York. (Perhaps this born and raised Southern Californian knew I'd get straight talk.)

Tuesday, March 17. Maybe I should've eaten some Lucky Charms cereal. At the clinic, the nurse practitioner looked at my underarm and breast, "It looks very suspicious." She continued, telling me she'd had breast cancer eight years ago, and had a mastectomy. I thought, *that may be your story, but it's not mine.* She scheduled my first mammogram for the following week at a nearby hospital. I was 44 years old. Mammograms were for women who had cancer, worried about cancer, or were hypochondriacs—especially if they had mammograms before age fifty.

After the clinic, I headed to the beach and walked—and walked. I had a little chat with God, "Use me. Let me know what I'm to do . . . ."

Just then a woman came running up to me, "Please help me! There's a beached baby seal; I need you to keep people away from it while I get the city workers."

The lady ran off and the seal started moving toward me—away from the ocean! "No. No baby. I'm not your mother! Oh geez!" When I got home I looked up what the seal totem represents: Listen to the inner voice. (The only inner voice I was willing to hear was saying this nurse practitioner was nuts!)

A week later, when the mammogram technician saw my breast, she went down the "this looks suspicious" road. Then *she* told me *she'd* had a mastectomy for breast cancer five years ago. I mused, "How strange." Women who've had breast cancer feel that everyone else has it, too. These are bumps in my underarm, and the breast looks a little different—but cancer? Give me a break! She looked at the films, then showed me areas of her concern before sending the results down the hall to the doctor. On my way out, she gave me a little bag of promo "goodies."

Unfazed, I asked, "Is this my 'boobie' prize?"

Next stop: Ultra sound. I lay there thinking, *The medical field looks for the bad until they find it.* After the ultra sound, the doctor came in, and in a soft, slow manner shared his opinion. I was furious. My inner logic yelled in private, *Turn on the lights and ask me to sit up, instead of my thinking there's a reason to remain laying in the dark for you and a technician to look down upon me!* The doctor

Chapter 1

began, "This doesn't look good." I just stared up at him. Slowly he asked, "Do-you-understand-what-I-just-said?"

The room still dark, I sat up. "Just because I'm not bawling my head off, doesn't mean I didn't hear or understand your point of view." I left in a huff. *They're off their rockers!*

I returned to church where I was working, then to the bank to deposit money for the church. In front of me stood a woman wearing a baseball cap, poorly covering her nearly baldhead. When she got to the bank teller window, I heard her say, "I just started chemo." In my mind I blessed her, then laughed to myself at the timing of the whole thing.

The following week, after church service, a woman visiting from out of town came to me for prayer. We prayed. Then she mentioned she'd had breast cancer years ago. Her comment caught me off guard. This is crazy! I studied her thin hair, and short, skimpy eyelashes, wondering what she looked like before. Before cancer . . . .

E-mail Updates

About every two weeks I'd send e-mail updates to select family and friends. As word got out, the list grew. Toward the end of treatment, I was updating fifteen to twenty people. I didn't try to hide my having cancer, but wasn't calling people with whom I'd been out of touch to inform them the news. To me, this was too intimate to treat like tabloid news for inquiring minds.

Allan: In 1997, I arrived in New Zealand for a three-month internship (which I managed to turn into an eighteen-month stay). Allan was my boss and boyfriend — then roommate and friend — then adversary. We returned to our friendship several years later — six months before my diagnosis.

Dear Allan,

Today everyone in the medical field who saw me used wording like, "This doesn't look good." "I hate to tell you this."

I'm not "phone ready" for anyone. I doubt they'll know anything before next week.

FYI to my knowledge, at this point only you, two other friends, and Mom and Dad are aware of what's been going on.

Thanks and xo, C

§

Hi, thanks for keeping me updated. I'll keep in touch this way until I hear differently. You know I'm not the type who can say that his prayers are with you but my thoughts are.

Cheers for now,

Allan

PS: Forgot to tell you but I hope you don't mind that I told Judith and both she and Gary are thinking of you. Gary said he even wants to give you a call which would be a nightmare since he is deaf as a post! He says the nicest things about you (Judith does too of course but it is newsworthy when Gary does). Cheers!

§

Michele: I met her as "Rosy the Clown" in 1989. I was completing an internship at a physical rehabilitation center. She had on a clown outfit, white face makeup and a tiny rose on the tip of her nose. When she approached me I told her I didn't like clowns. It seemed

Chapter 1

from that point on we'd show up at the same events, and eventually at each other's homes.

Dear Michele,

I got a call in the evening from the nurse practitioner. She just got a call from the guy who read my mammo films. The nurse canceled my appt with the doctor I was scheduled to see tomorrow morning. After talking with the guy who read the films, they felt I needed to skip tomorrow's appointment and meet with a surgeon—not someone who'd refer me to one.

So . . . now I've got a consultation with a surgeon on April 1. How funny. I'm getting the opportunity to laugh my ass off sooner than I thought! (April Fool's Day, in case you missed it.) Just don't book me for surgery on Good Friday—I've read the book.

Does this mean I should buy Easter Peeps now and let them "ripen" to stale stage, then eat them as a reward? I'm thinking that's a good idea!

xo,

C

§

buy the peeps, coat them in melted chocolate . . . no lumps, no bumps . . . coat them in colorful sprinkles, like confetti' and celebrate your brilliant health . . . chica

Michele

Tips for Him or Her:

✔ Share what's going on with someone you trust. Find a grounded, emotionally strong and supportive person. This is such a highly private, intimate and emotionally charged diagnosis. People can hardly say the word "cancer" let alone "breast," "nipple," "prostate," and "rectum." It's a crucial time to find how you, and others will cope.

✔ Consider bringing someone with you to the next few appointments. Even if you're strong, independent and quite capable—none of that's the point.

✔ Have someone be at home with you if they didn't come to the doctor's office.

✔ Don't run around telling the world you're having a biopsy. Some folks thrive on drama. They're the ones who'll tell you horror stories, warnings, and worry for you instead of providing strength. Choose wisely those with whom you share.

Tips for Those Who Want to Help:

✔ Bring them water if you see them in shock. Each time I hit the wall, on April 1, 7, and 23, someone got me water. It makes me laugh when I think of it. It's as if they didn't know what to do, so they did what they could—and maybe that's part of it. The act of compassion. And the water itself really did help me.

✔ Be there for them. Don't try to "fix" them.

Chapter 2

APRIL FOOL'S

Wednesday, April 1. Still thinking it was all a bit of joke, I had a biopsy at the same hospital where I'd had the mammogram and the ultrasound. (I actually thought I was showing up for a consultation—which in my mind was a "chat" with a doctor to straighten out all the unsolicited worry. Er . . . wrong. Joke's on me.)

This doctor immediately had me move out of the chair (I told you, I was there for a chat!) and onto the exam table. He asked, "What happened?" as if I'd run a red light and dented a car.

I requested clarification.

He tried again. "How'd you learn about the bumps in your underarm?"

"I saw and felt them."

Immediately he responded, "I think, as the films show—and everyone else feels—you have cancer."

Without checking how I was processing completely new information or pausing for questions, by rote he raced through the procedure of a mastectomy—cutting this, removing that. "Reconstruction three months later. Then in six months we'll add a nipple."

Huh? Whoa!

When he casually added, "It doesn't really hurt much," my initial judgment that this doctor was an old-school, pompous bastard solidified.

"You don't even have a biopsy, and in your mind you're doing a mastectomy on me? What will you do if you find out this is benign?"

He immediately, and frankly, answered, "The exact same thing."

My face flushed. Involuntarily, I shifted from my stonewall face to one of horror—I was still in disbelief, and now I mistrusted the doctor, too. Tears fell faster than I could wipe them away. He never even moved to look for a box of Kleenex, which was concealed behind him on the counter he'd leaned against.

He had me lie back on the exam table, then he called in a nurse and didn't introduce her. I couldn't see her at the head of the exam table. They performed a "punch" biopsy. It earns its name. I got a deep hole-punch with a cylinder four times in the breast. The second area punched wasn't completely numb. I yelped. He stopped to look at me, tears coming down my face again. "You okay?"

I flatly stated, "Yeah."

He carried on. When they were done, he patched me up, sat me up, and said, "Today is the hardest day." They left the exam room together.

Standing up I turned to get my bra, top, and purse hanging from the hook on the wall. Just below my clothes was the uncovered instrument table pooled with my dark blood. If my shaking hands didn't grasp my things correctly, they'd go splat—right into the blood, most likely splashing on me. I felt violated and ignored. I was very clear on where I wouldn't go for any further "care." I got dressed and stood in the room alone, shaking and crying. The reception area had been jam-packed when I arrived; *I better leave so someone else can have the room*, I thought.

Chapter 2

I moved forward from the shock I'd experienced in the exam room, stopping at the appointment desk on my way out. I stood there, crying tears of sadness and deep mistrust. The receptionist gave me a tissue and a small Dixie cup of water. The doctor reappeared in the hallway, and again stated, "Today is the hardest day."

I instructed him to phone me with the biopsy results. "If I don't answer, leave them on voicemail. I won't come back here for the results." He agreed to call me.

I sopped up my tears and pulled myself together to walk through the jam-packed waiting room. Empty! I had to laugh. Indeed. April Fool's Day.

Before I left, the receptionist handed me a hideous booklet on what to expect with a mastectomy. In my car, I fanned through it once before tossing it to the passenger floor. "Bullshit!"

It contained dated, scary drawings of an elderly woman in a bed, looking sorrowfully at her elderly husband, who looked dejected. More drawings, of an elderly woman with an IV in the hospital. My fear of being misdiagnosed erupted. As I drove home, a primal scream from depths I didn't know existed bellowed from within:

"NOOOOOOOO!"

It triggered tears to the extent I couldn't see the road. "God, help me. Bring to me the very best person to work for my highest good . . . ." I prayed out loud all the way home.

I put the booklet on the kitchen floor, face down next to the recycle can, questioning my keeping it, and questioning my tossing it out—which I did the following day.

I was in excruciating pain all day. Nothing had been suggested or given to me for pain, and Extra Strength Tylenol wasn't cutting it. Mom called. I couldn't stop sobbing. "Call the clinic that referred you. I'll call you back in two hours." It was 4:30 p.m. I called the clinic. The nurse practitioner was upset I'd not been completely numbed, and had me come in immediately. She gave me a strong prescription for the pain, then sent me to the pharmacy before it closed.

E-mail Updates

> *Obviously I'm not happy about the stress and upset that you are going through and I know it's easy for me to say, but I do think this is all going to work out okay. You'll come out the other side healthy and happy I'm sure. Keep these updates coming. Try to think generously of the medical people—they always do worst case scenarios as part of their job.*
>
> *Eat lots and have a beer with your mum.*
>
> *Catch ya soon.*
>
> *PS: Can you get someone to go with you to these appointments cos it's really good to have another person taking in the info.*
>
> *Allan*

§

> *i'm here with you and for you*
>
> *anything you want*
>
> *you got it*
>
> *be at peace*
>
> *love love love*
>
> *me and rosy . . . .*
>
> *Michele*

Chapter 2

§

Dear Allan,

Mom came up yesterday—she made veggie lasagna for me to freeze and take out as needed.

While Mom was here visiting, someone called from an oncologist (?) office connected to the biopsy doctor. (I didn't make the connection until I saw my mom's face.) They don't even have results yet and they're scheduling me! I made the appointment, stating I fully intended to cancel it Monday when I get the results. They immediately asked about insurance, etc. I told them I'd call on Monday with that info if they still needed it.

As for someone going with me to appointments—I thought this was going to be a consultation, a chat, not an invasion with blood left on the table two inches away from my purse and jacket.

I intend these e-mails to be more uplifting soon. Have a good tennis game this weekend.

C

PS: Below is part of an e-mail a friend sent—it just seemed to hit it right on:

[. . .] and i know

you know

there is a part of us that is totally blissfully beyond it

AND

there is the part that shouts

FUCK YOU AND THE WHITE HORSE YOU THINK YOU ARE RIDING

there is room for both

cry out loud

laugh out loud

love out loud

you are allowed

and

it will all get better

love love love . . . .

Michele

Chapter 2

Tips for Those Who Want to Help:

✔ Know your audience. Even if it's "just a biopsy," if your coping style is that of making jokes, tread very carefully. Overhearing my description two days after the biopsy, someone I love made a breast joke. Looking back, I see joking was his way of dealing with an issue he didn't understand, and he was trying to "lighten me up." It backfired.

✔ Have dinner made for the night of the biopsy. (Don't confuse this with taking them out for dinner.) They may be uncomfortable, and in a lot of fear. Not all biopsies are "punch" (think paper hole puncher to get a core of tissue). Another type of biopsy is "aspiration," using a needle. If the area worked upon is anesthetized, a biopsy is endurable. Even so, at minimum they'll have a needle injected into "that area."

✔ Offer to stay the night, if you don't live with them. You may be up all night listening to them—or listening to their silence. There can be strength in having a witness.

✔ Pray with them if you're both open to that. Or, just avoid expressing worry. Be a shoulder for them.

✔ Recognize your emotions. Fear, judgment, discomfort, pure love—you name it. Knowing where you really are with your emotions—not pretending or wishing, will help you.

✔ Offer a comforting touch, but realize when nerves are jangled, touching may not be welcome. The body may be on sensory overload.

Chapter 3

FROM OPTIMIST TO OSTRICH

I stopped at the beach to clear my head, hoping the doctor who'd taken the biopsy would leave a message on the phone while I was gone. As soon as I opened my front door, Ah! Voicemail. What relief. But it wasn't from the doctor. It was a vague message from the clinic, "Please give us a call to make an appointment for tomorrow morning to talk with the nurse practitioner." They've gotten some good news. (Did I tell you I was an optimist?) I called immediately. "I'm sorry. All I can tell you is the nurse wants to see you first thing tomorrow morning to talk about the results in person, and begin paperwork." This isn't even close to what I expected to hear. I'd gone from optimist to ostrich (head in the sand).

In the evening, purely by divine appointment, my good friend Mary dropped by and was on the couch when the biopsy doctor called.

"As we expected . . . . " He wanted to schedule a surgery date.

I had fully believed he'd say, "Wow. We sure were fooled. It's an infection!"

I thanked him for calling and said, "I'll be seeking a second opinion."

"That's fine, but don't waste any time."

I hung up the phone, looked over at Mary—and wailed. So sure of a mistake; now terrified that they weren't finding it. Mary offered to stay the night but I declined. "I'm so tired from crying, I'll sleep soundly."

E-mail Update

> *It is hard to know the right things to say. Read this cautiously and if it seems headed down a path you don't like then stop. It is inspired by your friend's comment re biggest balls. I have favorite poems or bits of poems and this is one bit from William Blake. It is very well known in England for reasons I'll explain sometime (yawn), is sung (commonly known as Jerusalem), and there's a movie that took its name from here. I have never read an analysis but it seems to be about summoning up the weapons (mental/spiritual) for a battle (mental/spiritual). It is defiant and says I've got the goods for this fight, bring it on.*
>
> *Bring me my bow of burning gold!*
>
> *Bring me my arrows of desire!*
>
> *Bring me my spear: Oh clouds unfold!*
>
> *Bring me my chariot of fire!*
>
> *I will not cease . . . .*
>
> *You have a bow of burning gold, arrows of desire, a chariot of fire.*
>
> *Allan*

Chapter 3

Tips for Him or Her:

✔ Get a second (or third) opinion, even if you like your first doctor. It's common, if not expected. You test out more than one car or pair of shoes, don't you?

✔ Ask people for opinions on the hospitals and doctors in your area.

✔ Ask each doctor what they believe your treatment plan will look like.

✔ Ask yourself how you feel about the doctor. Do they listen to you? Do they answer questions in a way you understand? What does your gut tell you?

✔ Look at the doctor biographies on the hospital website. Communication between doctors in the same hospital is assured with doctor rounds, where they talk about patient updates. It'll work to your advantage to have your doctors on the same treatment team.

✔ Stop doctor shopping once you've found your oncologist, surgical oncologist, and reconstructive surgeon. Do your homework beforehand, then be at peace with your choices.

✔ Exercise and meditate. These two nearly opposite approaches can help you deal with your emotions. Move your body. It'll help shake up the fear. Also, be still. If meditation is hard at this time, just sit in the silence for a few minutes throughout the day or when you can't sleep. On the inhale, feel the love. The peace. The strength. On the exhale, release the need to know, the need to control. Notice neither one of these approaches is analytical.

Tips for Those Who Want to Help:

✔ Be still. Be calm if you're around when a doctor calls. It's that quiet strength they'll anchor into while they're hearing news.

(When a doctor calls, it's usually not good news, unless it's a callback—from a question regarding a problem.) Stop background noise. It is up to you to move.

✔ Be ready to listen and comfort, not question or try to fix. Initiate contact. Ask what type of communication works best for them (text, e-mail, video chat, call, or card). It may change during the process.

✔ Know your audience. I met a woman who shared her husband's reaction to the news of her needing a mastectomy. "My husband said, 'Now we can wear the same swimsuits!'" I asked, "Are you still married to him?" She was taken aback, thinking I didn't understand—pointing to her breasts. She found his comment a comforting sign that he loved her no matter what her body looked like. I found his comment offensive.

✔ Throughout the process, let them know they're in your prayers or your thoughts—that they're loved. If that sort of language is tough for you, draw a smiley face on a piece of paper, or write "You're in my thoughts," or "I care about you." Bring them a tree leaf, flower, or sea shell. Something from your contact with Life.

✔ Don't be afraid to show your feelings, but make sure they aren't having to comfort you.

Chapter 4

AN APPOINTMENT WITH CHARLIE BROWN'S TEACHER

Tuesday, April 7. I sat in the clinic waiting room, fully dressed. The nurse practitioner came in.

"Receive any news?" she asked.

I reiterated what the doctor had said on the phone. She pulled out the results. Her New Yorker style was uncomplicated. "That's why I requested you to come in this morning. You have cancer." I listened to her. I looked right at her. I heard Charlie Brown's teacher.

She stopped. I imploded. Trembles crescendoed into convulsion-like shaking. Minutes later, tears quivered on the rim of my lower eyelids before plunging over, racing down my face. My body continued to violently shake. The nurse had someone bring me water.

"Do you need to lie down? Do you want sedation?"

"Like a dog going to the vet? No." I'd just completed my first year of self-employment, pouring money into the company rather than making it. I brought my tax return with me, per the clinic's request to show my income status. The nurse brought me back to the staff office and she filled out the forms for medical coverage. I've been covered for everything the whole way through, and I bless her every time I think of it. She then gave me the information I needed to call the cancer clinic and set up the appointment for my second opinion.

Okay God, if this is my path, and there's no way out but through, then you must provide me with people having the absolute best knowledge, talent, care, and compassion—while moving me through this with ease and grace. This was my prayer. My mantra. My answer.

E-mail Updates

Mike: We met in ministerial class. It was after lunch and the speaker for class was borrrring. Mike (MC) wrote me a note: *Toothpick?* I gave him a pack of dental floss from my purse. He sat shaking, stifling his laughter trying not to draw attention to us. He scribbled his second note: *To hold my eyes open!* He's now the senior minister of the Center for Spiritual Living, Granada Hills, CA.

> XXXXX MC *[This was Mike's entire e-mail. The font size he used was 40]*
>
> §
>
> Allan sent me the link to the YouTube video of Mario Lanza, "You'll Never Walk Alone."

Tips for Him or Her:

✔ Don't be around people who bring you down. This is where I had the benefit of living alone. I was really clear it was my time to heal, and if people weren't supportive, I either asked them not to call again, or the non-supportive event was evident enough to discontinue contact with each other. For me, these events came early on.

✔ Don't plan on getting support from "that person" later if you aren't getting it now. We can't make a cat act like a dog. You may need to rely on people outside your usual support circle for serenity.

✔ Immediately ask your doctor if they know of any state or federal programs to help with medical costs or getting insurance. If they don't know, ask where you can find the social worker or resource room.

✔ Ask if you qualify for financial aid. Begin filling out paperwork now. If you don't qualify, ask if they know of other programs. The following may help:

✔ Employment Development Department. Contact information varies from state to state.

✔ Social Security: Find your local office (1-800-772-1213) or www.socialsecurity.gov.

✔ American Cancer Society: 1-800-ACS-2345 (1-800-227-2345) or www.cancer.org.

✔ For medical and any other appointments, bring a pen and a pad of paper, and have questions written down ahead of time.

Chapter 5

REMORSE IN THE FROZEN FOOD AISLE

Thursday, April 23. The Cancer Clinic. My consultation for a second opinion with a surgical oncologist was moved up two weeks. I liked this surgeon. She was professional and compassionate, yet strong. I later learned she was one of the best surgical oncologists in Southern California—and the second person on my medical team from New York.

The information pelted down. "The largest tumor is 4.5 centimeters." "Stage 3." "Good prognosis with recommended treatment." "Currently a poor candidate for reconstruction." "Chemo may shrink the tumors . . . . "

Through my tears, discussion of options began, "What would you tell your best friend to do?"

"I'd insist they do chemo first, followed by a mastectomy, then we'd see what else."

"I'd planned to say no to chemo—and now surgery depends upon it?"

"If you say, 'no' to chemo, I can't operate. The tumor's so large in comparison to your breast size, not enough skin would be left to close-up your body. The reason for chemo before surgery is to shrink the tumor. Fifty to sixty percent of breast cancer patients have tumors partially shrink with chemo. Of those, twenty percent will have tumors shrink completely. But not everyone experiences tumor shrinkage. Ten percent will experience no change in size at all, and ten percent experience tumor growth with chemo."

Mine had to shrink.

"Come back with your answer at your follow-up appointment."

E-mail Updates
To: Bcc
April 23

> *Monday, April 27, I'll have a plastic surgery consult to see what he thinks are my options for reconstruction. I'm told he's renowned.*
>
> *Friday, May 1, Go for a CAT Scan to see if it has spread. I'll drink some stuff that morning so I'm super X-ray-able, so they can see EVERYTHING (including, apparently, if I need to poop!). Great.*
>
> *Monday, May 4, Meet with an oncologist.*
>
> *Wednesday, May 6, Another mammogram.*
>
> *Thursday, May 7, Another appointment with the surgical oncologist.*
>
> *Please do not call me with questions, or advice. I'm Soooo far from being OK with that.*
>
> *Thanks.*
>
> *I appreciate your love and support and knowing it's working out perfectly for me, quickly and with grace.*
>
> *Peace,*
>
> *Claudia*

§

> *Really appreciate updates though I know that's probably the last thing you could care about. Thanks. Allan*

Chapter 5

§

Good Morning my dear friend —

I didn't know what else to do . . . so I wrote you a prayer. (Imagine that!) I sent it as an attachment in case you weren't up for reading yet "another derned prayer!"

The timing of this must be unnerving. Just know that I, (and everyone who knows you. EVERY ONE OF US!!) love and support you! We will all be with you in Spirit today!

Thank-you for being my friend and in-spire-ation! I love you!
MC

§

—Hey there

You know you can't make a new alloy without some meltdown. You're just adding a little carbon to your steel.

I trust you're feeling better today.

Hang in there baby—and thanks for keeping in touch. I know it's not easy to do right now and I appreciate it.

Enjoy your beach day!

xxx,

MC

§

life is a yo yo

ups and downs

i'm with you in both

call me anytime

or come visit

love love love . . . .

Michele

§

Dear Michele,

To think last week I was freaking out over the thought of an implant—and now that's not even an option?!

Wow—I thought knees only knocked in cartoons!

§

Subject: yo ho ho

i would say ho ho ho and a bottle o rum, but i don't like rum

i don't like what is happening with you, either

I'm a port in this storm, for you both [my mom and me]

and i know all is well, and simple and beautiful

like you

Michele

I brought my answer to the follow-up appointment with the surgical oncologist (the one who would remove my breast and cancer). "I'll do chemo." Very pleased with my decision, she reiterated she couldn't recommend chemo more strongly. This would increase her ability to close me after surgery, although it came with no guarantee. Nor did it guarantee my becoming a good candidate for reconstruction. I told her I liked and trusted her. I'd see her again in a month, then again after completion of chemo for my pre-op appointment.

Chapter 5

I was keenly aware that since I'd agreed to chemo, I had to step into the game fully. I intended for the tumors to completely shrink. I would not bad-mouth chemo. I would not doubt it. I would see chemo as a blessing, fully doing its job.

I ate anything and everything I thought might taste good. That week, I ate a whole bag of potato chips, and half a bag of tortilla chips. Not bad for someone who didn't normally eat that sort of stuff! One day, I walked to the store early in the morning to get a banana as part of my breakfast. Ooooooh—a doughnut would be nice—Grabbed one! I got weepy as I passed the frozen chicken breasts, "Oh, I am so, so sorry."

The reconstruction consultation was the second and last appointment when I brought someone with me. Mom and I met up before heading to the appointment together. We rarely have arguments. The air was tense. I started off, "You're late."

"I know I'm late. Let's go."

She headed in one direction and I snapped, "The doctor's office is over here."

She pointed, "It's over there."

"Well, I'm going over here."

We eventually found the office. I loved this doctor right away. He came in without a white coat, and introduced himself by first and last name (which actually made me wonder if he was the doctor). As I read through my list of questions, he sat next to me to read the list with me. "If you'd shown up ten years ago with this size tumor, you would've been written off." He mentioned some chemo side effects: "Mouth sores, loss of taste, and loss of desire to eat."

I started crying. I'm 5'8" and weigh 116 pounds. "If I have a really tough time with it—" He understood I couldn't get through my sentence, "—We're not that pigheaded. We'd take you off." He was the third of four on my medical team from New York. I don't know what it was, but I found the New Yorker aspect comforting. He looked at my body (including down the back of my pants!) for where he'd get the skin for reconstructive surgery and realized there was no extra skin. When I expressed my concern of "robbing Peter to pay Paul" he said, "That's my job. That's what I do."

My mom and I came out of the appointment even more stressed out than when we went in. Our departure from each other was curt. The next day we talked. Mom shared that she cried for me as she drove home. I concurred, "I did too! I also cried for you, going through this with me. And for women in general—and for John." John is a man I met the previous October and cared for very deeply. He's a medical doctor who was then serving in rural Afghanistan. I decided not to share my news with him while he was over there. He'd return the following July. I felt it unfair to drop such news while he was in a war zone. He had a lag time of at least a month between his computer accesses.

E-mail Updates
To: Bcc
Date: April 27

> *Thanks for giving me space since the last update. I really appreciate it. I imagine I'll go in and out of needing space, and appreciate your understanding if I'm not up for calls, questions, etc. I'm finding I like shorter calls, and I'm OK with the silence, so please don't feel it's your job to fill in the quiet moments—I'd love to know you're sitting with me, holding the Light with/for me.*
>
> *My sister offered to be a skin donor—it won't work. I suggested a cadaver—it won't last.*
>
> *Bottom line: The tumor must shrink. That's that.*
>
> *The cancer clinic is new, clean and has friendly staff. It doesn't have the feel, look or smell of a hospital. The people I've seen don't look too bad.*

Chapter 5

What I know is that I've got an awesome group of people on my side! I'm in such gratitude for each of you.

Thanks for all your support and love.

With Love and Gratitude,

Claudia

Tips for Him or Her:

✔ Keep a list of names and numbers. Ask people to write down three concrete ideas of what they're willing to do. Have a friend call people on the list to set up dates and type of help. Will they help with holiday decorations? Will they drop by for fifteen to twenty minutes? Will they take you to appointments? Join you on a short walk? Take the kids somewhere?

✔ Realize you, the patient, are not the only one stressed out.

✔ Try to be gentle with loved ones, and strangers, too.

✔ Allow those around you time for their denial. They're going through what you've just completed. When I began sharing with people, one person screamed, "Nooooo!" Another person insisted my losing hair didn't have to happen. Their reaction came from love and shock and they were scrambling to make sense of it all. Positive thinking is one thing, but (with my back against the wall) I chose chemotherapy, and a very common side effect of chemo is hair loss. My prayers were for health, ease, and grace, and (usually) not outlining how it would happen like: ". . . . And I get to keep my hair."

✔ Be honest with yourself about your consciousness; your situation. For whatever reason, cancer showed up. There's always cause and effect. Take an honest look, then move forward. After my decision to take chemo, I was told of two work acquaintances who'd kept their cancer treatment 100% holistic. They both died that summer.

Tips for Those Who Want to Help:

✔ Worry won't change their diagnosis—and isn't good for you, either.

✔ Use music, nature, uplifting books, thoughts, and people to anchor you.

✔ Take walks, ride your bike, go surfing, climb a mountain—go into nature.

✔ Read something unrelated to cancer. Go to a light movie. Laugh.

✔ Scream songs that give you strength, make you happy, or fill your soul.

✔ Delve into your hobby—but if it's noisy or smells, run it by them first . . . .

✔ Do things that calm, restore, or exhilarate you.

✔ Have "me time" to better serve them.

✔ Send them supportive—not "get well"—cards and e-mails.

✔ Say to them: "I don't know what to say," "I wish I knew what to do," or "I wish I knew how to comfort you, or how to help you." These are all appropriate things to say to someone who's been diagnosed with cancer, or has a family member who's been diagnosed. The family members need support, too.

✔ Acknowledge their diagnosis of cancer while knowing that isn't their identity. It's okay to mention you're sorry they're going through this, and if you don't know what to say, say that. We express compassion when we hear someone's broken an arm, and the conversation doesn't drag on about it. Several people asked me if cancer was like having AIDS. I'm not sure, but the immune system is compromised, energy is low, and desire to eat is nearly gone. The best I could describe cancer in real terms for people was, "Think of the worst flu you ever had and multiply it many times over—never letting up for several months. A year later, barely having strength enough to lift 2.2 pounds (a liter of water) above waist height."

Chapter 6

STOCKING UP ON TOILET PAPER

E-mail Updates
To: Bcc
Date: May 1

>Today this cat got scanned . . . .
>
>By 8 a.m. I drank a 16 oz "berry flavored" barium drink (they call it barium because you think you're gonna die drinking that amount of what has the consistency of fresh cement). FYI—If you ever need to do this, drink it COLD, and with a straw!
>
>For the CAT Scan, I was taken to the "mobile unit" (a big semi truck in the parking lot that does more intense x-rays than what's in the hospital) and handed off to two men. We had a nice chat, then they found out I was new to this. They told me to drink a glass of water and lie down. As they put the dye into the I.V. they explained they'd be on the other side of the wall, but able to hear me. (Was that supposed to comfort me?) What I did find comforting was the sound of the machine while scanning me from shoulders to pelvis. It sounded like an airplane taking off!
>
>So, that's the skinny for today.

Thanks for your love and support,

Claudia

§

ah yes

i remember my scans well

and that was back in the 80s

hot dye pouring into my ruptured veins . . . they are just testing to see if you are

claustrophobic in those tubes

time never passed so slowly

but kiddo

you made it

another notch in your belt

you just have more knowledge and wisdom

to be a more complete minister

just my take

big love

P.S. i lost my hair too after my injury, and what i didn't lose . . . they shaved for surgery

show off that beautiful head

Michele

§

Dear Michele,

Yes! Hot dye, and right before they started up the machine they casually mention, "It will feel like you are actively urinating." WHAT?! This whole thing is so crazy! I'm

Chapter 6

not doing any more of this. They assured me, "You aren't—but women get this sensation." Sure enough.... Then I felt awful the rest of the day, which surprised me, as they just said drink water. I think it was the iodine? I'm not a big fan of shrimp. That's the only connection I can make.

I didn't know you lost your hair.

Love you.

C

I left my first oncology appointment with a boatload of prescriptions to relieve nausea. Wanting to barf at the whole idea, I opted to have the prescriptions filled another day. I finally got the nerve to ask, "Feeling nauseous, or actually throwing up?" I quickly remembered the wise advice, "Don't ask if you can't handle the answer." My lips quivered for four months. I never moved far from anti-nausea medication and I didn't engage in activities that promoted hurling, but I was fortunate: I never threw up!

Immediately after my appointment, I looked at wigs. It was to fulfill a dare I gave myself. I cried as soon as I saw the old-lady gray, unkempt wigs. I had beautiful, thick, wavy, mink-colored hair. I'd always loved everything about my hair. The wigs were u-g-l-y. The woman in the shop said, "I'm a survivor," which sped up my tears. I didn't want to associate with her, or the term "survivor." To me, survivor reeks of getting by, struggle, and enduring. Survivors (of anything) will tell you how tough they've had it, summing up their sad stories with, ". . . but I surrrviiived." I wanted out of the store. I'd fulfilled my dare.

That night I read about yet another surprise of cancer: When you lose your hair (especially if you have a lot of it) your head is extremely tender and itchy for the first day or two. (I'd never been bald. I was born 9 pounds, 4 ounces and looked like one of the Beatles, or Buddy Hackett.)

E-mail Updates
To: Bcc
Date: May 4

>Wow. I wonder when the shock stops. I guess when it's over.

>Today I met with an oncologist (a doctor who specializes in studying/working with people who have cancer). The one with whom I met was really sweet. Actually, TOO sweet for what I'd like. I felt I couldn't be real with her. I held back from verbally expressing most of my emotional shock with some things she told me—I felt she may call "code green" (patient out of control) if I swore or sobbed.

>They say I'm "Stage 3." It's Stage 3 because of the size and number of tumors. (Stage 4 is when people die and we ain't goin' there so don't get uptight.) The oncologist gave me her best sales job on chemo and drugs, then gave me some "statistics." After the numbers, I shared my math skills and memory of some tests, saying, "67% is a 'D'! Why on earth would someone aim for that?" I told her I'll do chemo because it'll allow them to close me up after surgery if (when) the tumors shrink. As for after-surgery drugs, I'm not sold on them at this point in time.

>Today meltdown #1: Learning there's another surgery—before chemo—to implant a chip that'll deliver chemo to (?) near (?) my heart (this is when I lost interest in listening).

>Meltdown #2: Hair loss. I've almost come to grips re: the wig—which I learned you don't get while you still have hair—it won't fit for when you don't have hair. So much to take in . . . I asked (doubt she would've shared without a direct question) "Eyebrows????" "Yes. They may go. Eyelashes, too."

Chapter 6

I stopped to see a social worker on the way out to talk about money. I mentioned what a disappointment this whole hair thing is. She gave me a flyer re: makeup classes! Cool!! I've never used an eyebrow pencil before!!

This week I'll have another blood draw, another mammogram, schedule an echocardiogram (they monitor the heart during chemo) look at wigs, fill out forms, remember how loved and supported I am—and eat everything I want because, get this—they say I may lose a taste for fresh veggies and fruit! I think that's when I shocked this oncologist with some 75 cent vocabulary.

Thanks for continuing to hold me in the Light.

With Love and Gratitude,

Claudia

§

yes, well it sucks what the physical body endures

this is where transcendence happens

faith is key operative

but keep informed

be spunky

be angry

let it go

go into the dark leviathan

your faith gets you out

hugs love faith

Michele

§

Karen: A great supervisor! We'd been out of touch and just after I was diagnosed, I received a note from her saying, "You've been on my mind. What's new?"

Dear Karen,

I guess now when people tell me to get lost, I'll say, "I can't, I've got this chip implanted." (I've spent my life avoiding things like chips in the name of health, and now a hospital is implanting one.) Actually, I called it a chip at the hospital and was corrected: "Port." Sheesh.

I know I'll come around, but right now I'm in the "cuss and cry" phase.

Happy Cinco de Mayo! Have a margarita and some CHIPS (not ports!)

xo,

C

§

Dear Claudia,

Thanks for the update. That was a lot of information to absorb. I wish I was closer to be of some support to you in your time of need. [Your siblings] are also supportive of you and what you are going through. No one knows what to say or how to say it to you because they fear you will lash out at them. Believe me, they are sympathetic, compassionate and understanding. They want to help you. There may come a time when you will need their help. Please don't shut them out of your life.

We all love you Claudia. We all want you to feel that you can talk with us and we will listen. Don't try to go

Chapter 6

through this alone. Cancer patients need family and friends to talk to and to listen to them. Know that we are all here for you.

This has been weighing heavily on our minds. I appreciate you sharing your progress with us. It is so difficult wading through all of the information as it is given to you. Do you bring a personal advocate with you during these consultations? If not, perhaps you should consider doing so as you may miss things that someone else can take notes and you can review later.

Love,

Dad

§

Dear Dad,

I think you may be missing some information in regard to how compassion and support have shown up thus far. I indeed have lashed out at those who've made jokes (protecting themselves from dealing with their emotions.) It's a wonder they're taken aback at mine being so raw. It has been less than a month since my diagnosis.

Let's talk.

Love,

C

 Before my second appointment with my oncologist, I called her.

 "I'd like to transfer doctors."

 I could tell she was taking it personally, so I shared my own experience of having had clients request to work with someone other than me. "I'd pair them with a better match, not taking offense," I told her.

A patient has an intimate relationship with his or her oncologist and nurse. In my case, I'll see the oncologist before chemo every two weeks for four months. Then every three months for a year after chemo; every six months for two years. Then yearly. "I appreciate your compassion, and that sweet baby photo on your lab coat says so much. I need a stronger presence. I felt I needed to monitor myself at my first appointment as you told me about the port, and my eyebrows. I didn't want to offend you, and I feared you couldn't deal with me goin' donkey leg." I even jokingly tried the breakup line, "It's not you. It's me." She didn't get it. I backpedaled. "This transfer request isn't about your skills; it's about our compatibility." She still didn't understand why I wanted to switch, which gave me an even stronger feeling I was doing the right thing. We agreed I'd stay with her two more visits until the oncologist I requested was back from vacation, meaning I'd begin chemo under her care before switching doctors.

That following Saturday evening, after eight hours of constant and increasing pain in my right axilla (armpit) where there were some small tumors, I called the on-call doctor. "I have an appointment with the oncologist Monday morning. I was trying to ride it out until then. Extra Strength Tylenol didn't touch the pain at noon, and the only other thing I have around is codeine, left over from the biopsy."

"Take that, and go to the emergency room if you still hurt when you wake up."

I awoke at 3 a.m. The thought of another thirty hours before seeing a doctor propelled me into action. I drove to the emergency room with my left arm. (I brought the right one with me too, but it didn't do any driving.)

I got in immediately. The ER doctor came in the room, exhausted. He listened while squatting to shift the weight on his tired feet. "I know the emergency room is a place for life and limb situations, but I didn't know what else to do with this pain for another day before my appointment."

Chapter 6

"Some people come in for stupid things. You're fine." Crying, I asked him if cancer was painful. "Some types." He maintained the tumor was putting pressure on the nerves in the axilla, creating pain, and encouraged me from here forward to take pain medication when I hurt (something I've always steered away from). "—And come back to the ER if needed."

So much goes on "behind the scenes" that I never imagined. I'm truly grateful for the love expressing in my life, and my medical team.

I'd become increasingly tired. I was good for about two hours, then needed a nap, and needed it now. Mom and I were out and I ended up taking a nap in the back seat of her car. She moved the car to a perfect spot just waiting for us. Under the shade of a tree in a quiet area of the parking lot, we rolled down the windows and opened a door for a delightful breeze. I was out fast for a good thirty minutes. When I got to my car I drove home, where I took a two-hour nap.

I wanted to keep my independence and live on my own, yet I knew I'd need help. The time was here. "Winding down to wind up." Time to surrender to the process. Not "white-flag" surrender, but to lean into God, and allow God to work through me— including working through the port and chemo as a healing agent. I knew I needed to approach it this way. I'd done my best making sure of no misdiagnosis. I wasn't about to be hacked into pieces, nor have chemicals dumped into me. Now I was making the decision to allow the healing to happen. I had no idea what I'd experience, or how the outcome would unfold, but it was time to move forward.

At the risk of giving too much information: For several days my system had been, shall we say, "clogged." Then I realized, well, geez! When you keep thinking of being "scared shitless" it's bound to show up that way!

Change your perspective about your experience with cancer. Change your vocabulary from war, battle, fight, struggle, victim, the big C, survivor, sick, and I have cancer to wording like condition, journey, I've been diagnosed with cancer, I had cancer, I went through the cancer experience. The idea is to state the fact without claiming having a disease (dis-ease). It's just a matter of changing your perception and semantics, and ultimately, consciousness. They play into our health and happiness.

Chapter 6

Tips for Him or Her:

✔ Stock up essentials before chemo begins (toilet paper, paper plates, etc. . . .) At this stage, I felt I had control in one area: Toilet paper. I kept buying it. Then I realized I had sixty-four double rolls!

✔ People will ask what type of food you like. Make sure you include things that count as liquids: Soup, puddings, fruit cups, juice.

✔ Let people know the list will change so they aren't buying you food in bulk.

✔ Stay clear of your favorite foods during chemo. Nothing tastes the same, and with nausea knocking at your door, the thought of "having seconds" of your once favorite food is gross. I craved food no one would've guessed. Roast beef and raw beef hot dogs for someone who hadn't eaten red meat in thirty years was the biggest shock. Also, ice cream and iceberg lettuce (no, not together), to give you an idea of healthy eating gone awry.

✔ Do what you can to focus on health, and ride with the tide for the rest.

✔ Have someone shopping with you handle the money, or use a debit or gift card instead of cash. It'll cut down on germs, time and thinking.

✔ Set up a special debit account with a minimal amount of money. The card can be given to those who run errands for you. Or, get a grocery gift card for your errand-runners to use.

✔ Read *Chemotherapy and You*, a 61 page gold mine from National Cancer Institute.

✔ National Cancer Institute. 1-800-4-CANCER (1-800-422-6237), or www.cancer.gov.

✔ Tell your doctors if you're in pain.

✔ Take pain medication when needed. Share any concerns about addiction with your medical team.

✔ Have paper towels for guests instead of hand towels in the bathroom. Use plastic utensils, disposable cups and paper plates. I hesitated on this, thinking about the environment. But with saving my energy and sanitation equating to health, it made sense. Think of it as saving water from not washing dishes.

✔ Try on wigs before chemo, but don't get one until you've lost your hair. It won't fit if you do. Many agencies or hospitals gift one wig. www.tlcdirect.org had some inexpensive, good looking wigs for women.

✔ Keep a gratitude list. It's all about perspective and gratitude. Be aware of all the good in your life: People, events and things. Keeping my list in view kept my focus on the good. Even when I felt rotten, my list helped me.

✔ Use sanitizer wipes or rubbing alcohol on anything shared: The refrigerator, microwave handle, phone, door knobs, kitchen cupboard knobs, light switches, counter tops, toilet flush handle . . . you get the idea.

✔ Get a small travel pillow. I kept mine next to the couch, under an end table. With the table skirt draping down, no one knew a pillow was there! I'd fold my blanket and put the pillow away after every use. It kept my place from looking or feeling like someone was "sick."

Tips for Those Who Want to Help:

✔ If you're a friend, ask how the family's doing. Offer them support.

✔ Take short walks or do light exercise with them, or their caretaker.

Chapter 6

✔ Take one day off work to help them, or their core support.

✔ Ask their preference, then pick up CDs, DVDs or books from the library.

✔ Offer to sit with them during chemo.

✔ Drive them to chemo or another appointment. There are so many. Lighten the load.

✔ Say so if you're okay with a call or trip to the emergency room any hour of night.

✔ Watch YouTube together; help her learn how to make a turban.

✔ Follow through on whatever you say you'll do.

✔ Stay in touch. Cancer can be an isolating experience.

✔ Be patient. They may lash out, or go silent—neither mean they don't need you. Their fear, anger, or confusion may get in the way of a normally happy, light, and loving personality.

✔ Be honest with them. Tell them if their new fear-based behavior is hurtful to you or others. They may not be aware of how they're coming across. If you're going to call them on this, be forewarned: Tender honesty works best; unconditional love is essential.

Chapter 7

A PORT IN THE STORM

E-mail Updates
To: Bcc
Date: May 7

Today I met with the surgical oncologist and we had a good, short meeting. She requested I get another biopsy today. Within minutes, a doctor from radiology came to get me. "Wow! She's not taking chances about my getting there!" On the way down the hall, the radiologist turned left; I turned right. I told him I felt a bit like a dog going to the vet. He laughed, "My dog is going to the vet today!" This guy was great. Real nice, calming, comforting. He and a coworker prepped and numbed me with epinephrine.

My heart began pounding then my body began shaking uncontrollably. First my left arm, then left leg; neck and head, followed by right arm, and right leg. It was a bit like the Hokey Pokey!—but all at once, and I didn't know what it was all about! My heart calmed down, then the shaking got worse. I was scared, "What's going on?" The radiologist who'd calmed me before said, "It seems the epinephrine may have gotten into your blood flow." My surgeon was brought in and the three of them suggested the emergency room. "No way." I finally stopped shaking. WILD!! I now was anesthetized from the epinephrine, so I suggested we continue with the biopsy. All three of them took a big "Mother May I" step backward.

The parking lot attendant was at lunch when I left, so the gate was open and that meant today's parking was FREE!!!

Thanks for your support.

With Love and Gratitude,

Claudia

§

i know

my change happened fast too

but i was out of it

i was in icu for 3 months

yours is different

you have to face this life event more

full on

choices, awareness

sometimes I'm afraid for you

and then

i see you

beautiful, enlightened and, enriched

this is a tough road chica

I'm your shoulder

Michele

Chapter 7

§

Cathy: My sister. She immediately offered help, and was a bit put out when I wasn't jumping for it. I had no idea what needed to be done. I was in "deer in headlight" pose.

> *Dear Cathy,*
>
> *I appreciate your offer for help. Right now I'm getting things in order—not really knowing what to expect. It takes everything we associate with being feminine: the hair—including eyebrows—the period, then the breast. Jeepers Creepers. But somehow we just move forward.*
>
> *Love you,*
>
> *C*

§

> *Again, let me know what you need to get things ready and if I can help. On the delicate subject, my not knowing what to expect for you and how to help. Please let me know what will be best for you. If you need me to drive you somewhere, or pick up something or research things. I won't know unless you tell me. I've heard of make over classes to keep you cute and sassy looking. Maybe we can do that. Are there colors you are finding yourself drawn to?*
>
> *Lots of love,*
>
> *Cathy*

§

> *Dear Cathy,*
>
> *Driving may be something I need later on. I dread you or Mom having to drive fifty miles each way, then, driving me another twenty miles each way to take me to the clinic or hospital.*

Yes, it is a delicate subject right now—and may be the whole way through. I swing from really good perspective to not so great throughout the day.

I do know I'll need people to hold back laughing at me and making jokes at my expense. In the past, that hasn't been a strong suit of my siblings. (My questionable swimming skills into adulthood, Italian/Scandinavian gene of blonde, hairy arms as a kid, and the biopsy. At all times I was giving it my best.) I also need people around me who are okay with my crying, but who don't feel sorry for me. I'm switching oncologists because I don't feel her strength. I need people around me who are strong. I send updates to some people. Just not sure who I want on board with me yet.

I tried on wigs the other day. It's not just slapping on a wig like when I was a kid wearing Mom's long blonde one. Everything seems to be more hassle than it appears— scarves, makeup, hats. So much to learn.

Love,

C

§

Dear Claudia,

I liked the message you sent out yesterday. It was very positive. My suggestion is to plan your future hospital trips so you leave while the parking lot guy is out to lunch.

I hope things go well with radiology on Monday as they talk about the port placement procedure.

It is now 6:20 p.m. and we just got back from church. I thought about you during the service. I'm not a religious person Claudia but I did pray for you as I do every night *after I turn out the light before going to sleep. I asked God to see you through this crisis in your life. I told God that I would gladly change places with you. I'm almost seventy-eight-years-old and have had a long and good life. I would gladly die if he would heal you of your cancer.*

I love you!

Dad

§

Dear Dad,

Whoa—so much to touch on in this e-mail. It may come over a few e-mails.

First, I don't believe God sees this as a crisis. I'd love—whether you pray or not—if you know in your heart and mind, that I'm healthy. I'm not sharing this journey with people who get stuck in worry. That doesn't help me—or anyone else.

I don't believe God "makes deals"—and I'd lose my faith if God would change places of individuals in a situation like this. I'm not afraid of death, I'm just really scared of this process—much of it being "the unknown."

I've got a strong feeling when this is over it'll help me help others—whether as a licensed minister or not. I'm a strong, independent lady and people respect me for how I've gone through life.

I don't believe God is on a cloud making choices, "You get; you don't." I believe God is more of an energy that works for our good, and responds to our direction (that's why focusing on the positive is so important). Sometimes God shows up as lessons (not tests). This may help me fulfill my purpose as a life teacher, I don't know. I may never know—so for now, I just move forward.

I love you and would never wish this on you—or anyone. I'll get through it. Just with lots of tears—and they'll end one day. I've got a great medical team.

I love you!

C

§

E-Mails
To: Bcc
Date: May 10

When they mentioned PORT, I thought SHIP, or WINE.

Had a port consult today. It was the first appointment where I didn't have to take off my clothes, give blood, or get stabbed. So, yes, it went well.

Terminology: PORT—It's a "little" gizmo they implant into the chest that has a quarter-size thing on one end (about five stacked quarters in height) and a wire that comes out of it. (Think miniature computer mouse.) The wire goes to the heart via a vein. After scraping me up from the floor after the description of the procedure, they said it's the safest, most comfortable option, and has the fewest complications and can come out after chemo.

My concern then quickly moved to scarring. Where, how big, geez—another scar. They looked up who the scheduled surgeon was, and laughed. This guy specialized in plastic surgery before he switched over to this department. They assured me he's my best bet for beautiful outcome as a bonus.

The purpose of a port is to avoid being stabbed in the arm for tests, chemo etc, and damaging veins. I thought they'd

Chapter 7

just plug me in. But no, they'll still stab me—just in the chest, not the arm. Hmmmm . . . Progress??

I'll have this "placement" as they call it ("implant" is what it seems like) on May 27th. Then they'll have me go without a shower for 4 days, and if I'm still smiling, I begin chemo.

This Friday I've got an echocardiogram (an ultrasound of my heart).

Next Monday I've got an appointment with the oncologist I'm transferring from. I'll be under her care until the third week in June, when my new oncologist returns from vacation. (What—did they tell him, "Mulcahy's not a lightweight—I suggest you take your vacation before taking her on"?)

Thanks for continuing to see me as healthy and happy.

xo

God's Peace,

Claudia

§

I'm not going away so don't worry if I seem to drift off at times. I know you'll be surprised when I tell you that I just get wrapped up totally in my own things from time to time. From now to 29/6 (exam) I'll be doing heaps of study.

Catch ya,

Allan

§

Dear Allan,

No worries. I haven't become high maintenance.

§

Dear Karen,

I've decided this whole thing is B.S. I suspected it before, but now it's confirmed. I just felt I was making friends with the whole gig—then the phone rang. It was the chemo people. "Be here June 3rd at 8:00 a.m.—for SIX hours!!! Uh, was that in the small print?!" As for pain, I'm OK. I've got meds—and I know how to use them! I'm just not lifting my arm (DON'T WAVE TO ME!!)

Keep the peace, baby,

C

§

Well, this is a welcome message! I've been reluctant to call cuz I always seem to say stuff that upsets you. That is not my intent! You're in the prayer circle and in my prayers.

By the tone of your e-mails, it sounds like you're finding your way around OK—in spite of all "the stuff." I'm not surprised . . . you do have a "mighty consciousness" after all! I should be so brave! Puts my petty BS into perspective.

Speaking of petty BS . . . I signed up for a ten-day silent retreat in Central CA for the first week in July (I mean it's not like I don't have any work to do right now!) My intention is to purge the pettiness! I think you have a pretty good idea what that is for me . . . . Now it's my turn to find out!

Take care of yourself my friend. Know that you are in my thoughts daily.

Peace, Blessings, and warmest regards!

love, MC

Chapter 7

§

when they said port

you thought they said snort

guffaw, chuckle

well, it sounds . . . medical

and medically sound

yeah, i remember morphine and nausea

heaven and hell

you go girly girl

the force of Zena is with you

big love

Michele

Friday, May 29. Port placement. The operating room nurse prepped me for surgery. The assisting surgeon, Dr. Wurm (as in worm) gave me the rundown of what would happen during surgery. I met my attending surgeon, Dr. Finch (as in bird) while I lay on the operating table. I'd been forewarned, "He's a bit cagey but a great surgeon, and great with esthetics."

Sizing me up, the surgeon shared the same out-loud thought as every doctor has in this process, "You're very thin. We could use a 'petite port'—it's used for 'emaciated males.' You'll still feel the skin stretch. There's just no fat on your chest to go over the bump of the port. You'll be awake during the procedure, but not care about anything."

I go into any procedure or surgery verbally thanking those involved for being there, and for being on their "Top Game." Then, I silently bless everyone, including me as I fade off. This time I was conscious and blissed-out during the two hour procedure and the rest of the day. (Thanks to valium, morphine, and a cherry on top—anti-nausea medication!)

Leaving the surgery, I told the nurse who'd forewarned about my surgeon's demeanor, "Dr. Finch was terrific." The nurse gave me a blank stare. "Really. After the procedure I thanked him. He gave me a smile, thumbs-up, and said, 'You did great.'" The nurse laughed at how social that was of my "cagey" surgeon.

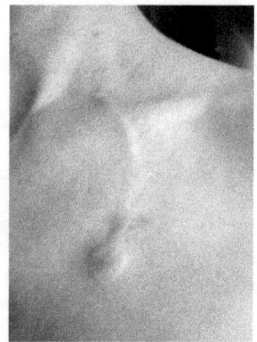 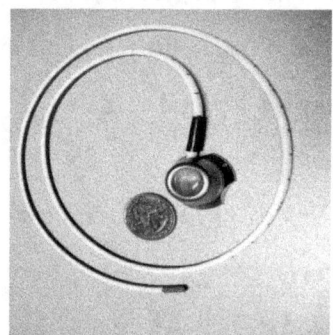

My petite port   *The standard port*

The standard port is the size of a quarter, about five quarters in height. The protruding part is called a button (where they administer the chemo). A small hole was made in my neck so they could thread the wire through a vein from the port to my heart, then back down, making a loop. The port can be removed when cancer treatment is over. Surgery is followed by four days of changing bandages and keeping the site dry. The bit about, "You'll feel your skin stretch over this"—Now I understand!

I stayed at Mom's for four days. On the third evening I announced, "Wow, I'm healing fast! I can feel the skin beginning to itch a little bit." I gently ran my fingers over the bandage to satisfy the itch. "WHOA!" Not so fast, kiddo! Obviously not ready for that trick! Healing is one thing, showing off is another. The port site remained tender for several weeks.

I still had chest pain five days after the port placement. I called the on-call radiologist to ask about the excruciating pain to bend,

Chapter 7

lie, breathe deeply, or laugh. "It's like swallowing a piece of an apple the wrong way." They knew exactly what I meant. "It's because you're thin and the port doesn't have any fat to snuggle into. But it's a good sign that you're healing. The body is recognizing your new friend." Man, I've got new friends everywhere!

Tips for Him or Her:

✔ Make a list of birthdays and holidays before each round of chemo, if sending cards to others is important to you. After my first treatment, I realized I forgot to call my friend Allan on his birthday. He called me and couldn't understand why I was apologizing. He'd received a birthday card I'd written and sent earlier! The card system worked. I began writing out birthday cards for the next month.

✔ Ask people to continue reaching out—to initiate contact; to follow through. If they say, "I've been meaning to . . ." (send a card, call, drop by) call them on it. Help them help you.

Tips for Those Who Want to Help:

✔ Include them. Invite them to activities. Let them decide if they're able or not to attend.

✔ Pass information on to them. If people mention to you "They're in my prayers," "How is she?" "Send him my love"—Share it! Hearing these reminders is like following breadcrumbs on the healing path. My mom told her water deliveryman about me, and with every delivery she'd relay his greetings. I also got cards from people I didn't know. These weren't only blessings to me, they supported my mom as well.

✔ Tell him or her about Certified Hypnotherapist Brennan Smith: www.BrennanSmith.com. I used his hypnotherapy downloads daily for pain reduction, tumor-shrinking visualization, and deep, peaceful sleep.

Chapter 8

HOW SPIRIT SHOWED UP FOR ME

Walking a path of spirituality doesn't mean we don't have things to heal, or that tough situations won't happen. It can mean we have an opportunity get out of our own way, and move through the situation with ease, grace, and more awareness. Walking a path of spirituality doesn't mean having it all together. That's like eating once and for all. Be gentle with yourself. God is not "testing" you, nor is this punishment. You may never know the reason "why." We've all got our stuff to heal. Some issues are just more visible— but we've all got our stuff.

§

The week of diagnosis, four complete strangers complimented me without knowing what was going on in my world. They talked about things I wouldn't lose from cancer. "What a great sense of color and style you have." "You have the most beautiful eyes." "You can get anything with that smile. Anything. What a beautiful smile!" This from a guy at the Can and Bottle Recycle on April 16. He let me go ahead in line. I thanked him. His compliment about my smile was just what I needed to hear—then I began to cry. Taken aback, he exclaimed, "What? Did you pay your taxes yesterday?"

I surprised myself, sharing my news with him. He had genuine compassion and gave me a gentle, but sincere hug. "I don't know why I'm telling you this, but I work across the street"—pointing to a Catholic elementary school—"I'll say a prayer for you. God bless you."

"God does bless me. I'm a bit pissed off right now—but God does bless me."

He grinned and nodded, "What you are feeling is normal. Be okay with that."

The following week I had enough energy to make some lemon bars and I took them over to the school office. "This is going to sound really strange."

They laughed. "We've heard it all."

"Okay. I met this man who works here. He had on shorts, and is about this tall."

"Oh! That's one of our two male teachers! Bob, the P.E. Coach." They looked all over for him but he was gone. I left the lemon squares. I felt comfort knowing an angel worked just a block away from my apartment.

The Universe supports us. If we're open, we'll see the support everywhere. Spirit worked through these people, letting me know I wouldn't walk alone. We never know what's going on in the lives of those around us. My experiences from these encounters with strangers were reminders that Spirit works in, around, through and for us.

§

I woke up with the song, "You'll never walk alone" on my mind. An omen to the day's unfolding of events. At 8 a.m. I called the Employment Development Department to inquire about a form the social worker gave me. I was self-employed, and a contract employee at church—I hadn't been paying into disability. I didn't qualify for benefits. I asked the young man on the phone if he might

Chapter 8

know of any other programs for which I might qualify. He asked, "Did you get injured on the job? Is this an injury that requires you to seek a new job?"

I said, "Cancer." (Noticing I left out "I have").

"Oh—" Fully expecting him to complete his reflection with something like, "My grandmother had cancer." But instead, he knocked me off my chair. "This isn't a state number, but you may want to call them to see if they can help: 1-800-ACS-2345. I volunteer for the American Cancer Society. That's their number." It's not even 8:05 a.m. and manna has shown up in the bureaucracy of calls and paperwork!

§

During this first month (April 7–May 7) there was a recurring scene I kept getting in my thoughts and feelings. It was an energy that felt male, clear, strong, and safe. I saw flashes of an image a few times, and I recognized it as Jesus. He usually stood behind me on my left side, but sometimes sat in front and to the right. I would hear a strong, compassionate voice, with the same words every time, "It seems so real, doesn't it?" Wow—this really does seem so crazy-real! That blip comforted me, anchored me. Then I was conscious of me and my box of Kleenex on the couch again.

Things like cancer are an experience the soul is having as a human. Try not to get lost in it.

§

I also felt the energy of a hand on my left shoulder and recognized it as Lucille, a dear friend of mine who was spiritually and mentally strong, beautiful, and my mentor in so many ways. She'd died a few years earlier, at age ninety-four. At other times, I could hear her command, "You can do this!"—with frustration at my hesitancy some days.

§

My schedule was filled with medical appointments three to four times a week. Almost every time on my travels to the cancer clinic, I'd see red-tailed hawks flying. I got a hit of strength seeing them. In that moment I "got it." This was my journey, not my destination.

The hawk totem represents a message: Step back. Get a bigger view versus a narrow focus. Keep the analytical mind under control, not allowing it to run wild. The hawk usually means hard work is involved, with great rewards.

§

I agreed to present a section at a workshop for women. I began, "We're going on a guided meditation." A latecomer entered the room. I could see plastic tubes, and gauze patches hanging out of her tank top. My heart started pounding. She pulled up a chair directly across from me in the circle while apologizing for being late, "I recently had a mastectomy. I got a slow start today." For the first time, I put two-and-two together, figuring God was showing me all these "coincidences" in bits and pieces to prepare me.

Thy will be done, not my will. We cannot force things into existence or nonexistence. I was beginning to entertain the thought that just perhaps God had been showing me through the clinic, hospital, bank, church, and again at this workshop I'd be okay; I'd be carried. Like the poem, *Footprints*—"During your times of trial and suffering, when you see only one set of footprints, it was then that I carried you."

§

My friend Brennan, a hypnotherapist, sent me three download sessions he created for me. I listened to them daily. I had a recurring scene come to me: I was in a pool learning to float on my back, leaning my head back into big hands I trusted. (Sometimes they looked like large, white wings.) I felt comforted, like I was surrounded by a soft blanket, or angel wings.

A month later I had another image—even stronger than the one with me in the pool resting my head in wings. This time, I was floating on my back, perpendicular to the flow of a river. I'd get midpoint when the water became really rough: ocean-like, splashing over my face, tossing me about. In this meditation, I'd see one of those lifesaving poles you find near a pool. Then, I'd feel that pole under my upper back, neck and head. I'd be guided and pulled to shore. I'd hear, "Trust. Float." And I'd see a crowd of people on the shore, waiting for me. In subsequent meditations, the crowd grew.

These images were so comforting to me. I could see and feel through my fear and rough water, I am—and will be—taken care of. I spent many years overcoming fear of water. I'm still not a strong swimmer, but I can enjoy swimming in a pool, and boogie boarding or snorkeling in the ocean. I find it interesting that now, the images of safety, comfort and strength are water based. I guess that's how I know the Spirit is doing the work. I overcame the fear of water; now water is where I find my strength. Metaphysically, water represents consciousness.

§

There's a story I remember from years ago that my minister, Marilyn, at that time shared in her sermon. The story is about a man who had a son. Everyone said, "You're so fortunate to have a son." One day the son was given a beautiful horse as a gift from a friend. Everyone said, "You're so fortunate, your son has been given such a fabulous horse." The son fell off the horse. He broke his arms, and legs. Everyone said, "This is terrible! Your son has fallen off his horse and broken both his arms and legs. How awful!"

The father said, "Judging, judging, you are always judging."

The king's army came through the village to collect all the young men and take them into a war everyone knew they would lose. This boy wasn't taken because of his broken arms and legs. Everyone said, "How lucky you are that they did not take your son!"

The father said, "Judging, judging, you are always judging."

§

We don't know why certain things happen the way they do. Maybe it's a gift in some wild wrapping! Go easy on judgment.

Chapter 9

GOD THROWS A PARTY

AFTER CHEMO #1 (WEEKS ONE AND TWO)

The game is to keep food in your stomach—but not too much. You won't be eating the same amount you did before chemo. Eat like a bird—often, and one peck at a time.

I ate anything I desired. (Mind you, the list was pretty short!) The evening following each chemo, my dinner was half a cup of room temperature chicken broth, some saltine crackers and 7-Up. A few days later, I craved macaroni and cheese, and it had to be Kraft. At first, I couldn't get enough Gatorade. Now I hate it, as I do garlic, chicken broth and saltine crackers. I ate one watermelon a week! And I still like it! Other than craving vanilla ice cream (I managed to go through one half-gallon a month for four months!) I lost desire for sugar. My stale Easter Bunny Peeps safely peered over the rip in their cellophane window.

Here are foods that worked for me after the first chemo:

Carrot soup (tepid), chicken broth (tepid), saltine crackers. Hot dog (straight from the fridge). Instant pudding. String cheese, mac and cheese (tepid). Boiled potato (tepid, with a bit of honey mustard salad dressing). Scrambled egg (nothing added, not even milk or water). Nectarines, bananas, apples. Don't like prunes? Eat 'em anyway.

Crazy. I'd been looking forward to the "Look Good, Feel Better" class. It kept me from thinking of other upcoming things. After class the port would get its first use for what they call a "fast port draw." (Hmm . . . a really quick portrait?). No, blood work taken from the port, rather than the arm. Two days later I'd have my first chemo treatment. I had that "dog going to the vet" feeling again.

With a little bit of knowledge and practice, the makeup class proved to me I could actually look great. A big thanks to the volunteers teaching this class, and to the companies donating the makeup. Because of the risk of infection from bacteria, American Cancer Society highly suggests getting rid of all currently used makeup. Get plenty of Q-tips and cotton balls. Get rid of sponges and makeup brushes. Wipe off lipstick after each use. No "double dipping" into anything—not even pumping air into mascara. I was able to use mascara for about a month before losing my eyelashes and implementing the tricks they taught in this class that minimized the obvious lack of eyelashes, eyebrows, and face color. Yes, naps come shortly after makeup is on. Why do you think they call her Sleeping Beauty?

In addition to learning how to apply makeup in this class, I got to try on wigs and scarves for color and style. One of the women thought my wig was so real looking. I didn't have a wig! I was the only one in the class of six who hadn't begun chemo. Christine, the woman who liked my "wig" invited me to come to her place the following day to try on wigs. She even lent me one. Christine drove, cooked and did things. I was relieved and impressed to see how life would continue during chemo. I later learned she'd been on a break for a few months between her chemo treatments!

The morning of my first day of chemo, my period began. The last one ended 15 days earlier. I am woman! During my first appointment with my first oncologist, she informed me my menstrual cycle would stop during chemo, and because I was 44, it most likely wouldn't start again. I stood at my doorway, ready to

Chapter 9

leave, thinking: As much as having a period can propel you to feel ugly, bloated, sleepy, cranky and some days sad, it's a gift. Oh brother, now she's getting sentimental over saying goodbye to another "friend"! But realizing my sewing days were over, (I can't "mend-straight" anymore!) I felt a bit of sadness about this loss—one more feminine aspect taken from me on this journey: My hair, my breast, my menstrual cycle. Perhaps it's one less thing to be concerned with while traveling. The whole situation reminded me of Shakespeare's Twelfth Night:

"Some are born great. Some are made great. Some are thrust into greatness."

I got to the point where I fully decided to see chemo as my friend. With chemo, the tumors were expected to shrink, allowing for an even more successful surgery and reconstruction. The idea with chemo, really, is to bring one as close to death as possible, to give one life. (For whoever wishes to save his life will lose it, and whoever loses his life for my sake and the sake of my gospel will save it. Mark 8:35) Not exactly what I had in mind.

I'd have two types of chemo. My oncologist said the first two months will be the roughest. Every two weeks I'd have my blood drawn to monitor my white blood cell levels. The following day, I'd receive Adriamycin and Cytoxan chemo, and the day after that I'd go back to the clinic for a shot. (Vodka anyone?) The injection of Neupogen into my stomach would stimulate white blood cell production to boost the immune system, which becomes more compromised as chemo treatments progress.

I'd switch over to Taxol (the second type of chemo) for months three and four. Again, preceded with a blood test, and followed with a different injection, Neulasta, to help prevent infection. White blood cells are fast growing and fight infection. Chemo kills all fast growing cells—both good and bad. Having a low white blood cell count is called neutropenia.

With each blood draw and chemo treatment, the port is wiped clean with alcohol. An extension catheter is plugged (more like poked) with a needle into the port, which waits to receive the catheter delivering the chemo. The nurse dons protective gear, hangs the bag marked "Hazardous Material" to the I.V., then connects it to a catheter leading to the port. Two nurses would come in the room and ask me to say my full name, birthdate and what type of chemo I was receiving. They cross check my current weight, white blood cell count, and the amount of chemo I'd receive that day. My treatments tended to last five hours. Day one, on the way to the restroom with my I.V. rolling along side of me, I received shocking news about Adriamycin: "You'll have red urine the first few times. After Cytoxan, it's blue!"

E-mail Updates

>*Dear Karen,*
>
>*Again, my timing was off for the tours given at the Cancer Clinic. Frustrated and scared from missing the tours, I explained my situation to a woman at the reception desk, crying as soon as I began to talk. The woman came out from behind the desk and hugged me, then took my hand and walked me to the chemo area. (I said I needed to see it before my first chemo in two days.) I felt like a kindergartner on my first day of school, but I left feeling better. Much better.*

To: Bcc
Date: June 4

>*I love my hair. My smile. My eyebrows. My teeth. My weight. My neck. And I love you. You are all on my "Wall of Gratitude." So are shade trees and Kleenex.*
>
>*Going over check list for the millionth time before leaving the house to meet my new friend, chemo.*

Chapter 9

Carpet vacuumed, mirrors clean, bills paid, washed or ironed just about everything. Bed made, plants watered, car washed. Have supplies like moisturizing toothpaste, toilet paper, paper towels, paper plates, plastic utensils. I was told cotton scarves stay in place. I've got more than fifteen scarves—all silk or nylon! So I bought a large cotton scarf (35 inch, square) and a T-shirt, and now must learn to make turbans.

MANY thanks to my mom who did most of the shopping because the port placement caused pain longer than we expected.

Well, lunch is made, medications packed, prayers said, driver's waiting . . . .

Mary drove me. We arrived in the clinic parking lot and sat for a few minutes, not talking. Just sitting in peace, in the morning sunshine. Then tears slowly glided down my face without my obstructing them. We remained sitting in silence. A few clouds moved in overhead. When I stopped crying, I was ready to go in. The sky opened up making way for big, fat, raindrops! I like to think it was my angels and other Spirit guides, letting me know they were aware of my fear—yet the rain wasn't their tears, but sort of confetti that I was moving forward and all is—and will be—well. As we got out of the car, it rained harder and faster and was really cold rain! I ran toward the building. A man passing by asked, "Who started this?" I said, "I did!" He looked at me and laughed. About 15 minutes later, we could hear hail pinging against the windows. (That must've been God celebrating when I sat in the chair for chemo!)

Ready-Set-Go! "Saline, Saline, Over the deep blue sea . . . ." They flush the port with saline before beginning chemo.

The chairs were lined up somewhat resembling a beauty salon. While I was being hooked up to an I.V., there were five researchers in the small space next to me with only a curtain between us. They were loud, and not aware of the doom and gloom they spread. I mentioned to the nurse it was my first day, and I was listening to an Iyanla Van Zant Giving Thanks CD on my iPod to get into the right frame of mind for my healing to take place. The instructions I'd received were: Bring in only one friend, no kids and to be mindful of any TV or cell phone volume. Within ten minutes I was moved to a private room with a sliding glass door. It was bigger, quieter, and I had a bed! "Your preference for a private room will be heard, but there's no promise you'll get it. It's for those having chemo treatments over five hours, and for those with back problems." OK, I've never pulled this card before, but I said, "For what it's worth, I've got a spine fusion with a 13-inch rod."

I chatted a bit with Mary, fell asleep, and then I had a visitor, the woman who befriended me in the makeup class. Christine and I had similar chemo schedules and knowing it was my first day, she was walking around with her I.V. looking for me. It was great to see her! She's on a different type of chemo. It's easier on her body and her sessions are shorter, but she's on it for a longer period of time, perhaps life.

Mary was a great chemo guest. She'd go to the pharmacy for me, get me juice, read through the "what to expect" piles of paper, and stayed at my place on chemo night. She read some pages out loud from Emmet Fox, made my meals (which are very small but frequent.) She's great about hygiene to the degree I've never had to think of before. (Using paper towels, bringing her own towels, toothpaste, etc.)

Chapter 9

It's Thursday. Tonight I'm on my own. I asked my manager to check on me tomorrow. She came by today while Mary was here. I was sleeping. She'll come by again Friday.

That's the skinny for this week. Got the immune shot today and have been sneezing since! (Achoo! God Bless Me!!!)

Much love,

C

Already, my naps were consistently two hours long. When I woke up, I'd eat a raw hot dog right out of the refrigerator. What the heck were hot dogs doing in my refrigerator? Ah, yes, the taste buds were already changing!

Mom came up Saturday. She was getting ready to leave that night and I stood there crying, afraid of what would happen in the morning. She asked me if I wanted her to stay the night. My energy was low and pain high from the port placement. My hair was already brittle. I couldn't cope with the idea of a chunk of hair falling out this early on. Mom stayed, "sleeping" on an air mattress. The set up was absolutely hysterical. I directed her where to find the mattress, how to go about inflating it and closing the valve before all the air flew out. This was a ridiculous request of mine that my then seventy-eight-year-old mom fulfilled. If I hadn't been in pain from the port, it would've been fun. We'd laugh, then I'd be in pain from laughing, so we'd be serious—then we'd laugh from being so serious!

Mom fulfilled my requests. She made hard-boiled eggs, "Blue Box" mac and cheese, and instant pudding. If you knew my mom and her cooking skills, you would know this was all a bit of a joke—from box to paper plate. Not her style! I think she couldn't stand it. She made some homemade soup "to have on hand." The joke at the local Vons grocery store was I'd become a four-year-old's best friend with my new food cravings. The managers where I live are great! I asked them to peek into the window when they walked by if they hadn't seen me around. They kept a look out for me. What a huge relief: Getting my mail on days I didn't make it to the mailbox and making one-item trips to the store for me. The maintenance crew took my trash to the dumpster when I put a bag on my doorstep.

Between January and March that year I had four neighbors with whom I was close—each moved out of state. In April, the time of my diagnosis, there were four empty apartments around me. New upstairs neighbors moved in the week I got my port. Their bedtime was between midnight and 2 a.m.. They were heavy footed, smokers, young, and noisy. They were unemployed and homebodies—meaning all of us were home all the time.

The maintenance crew thought they'd fixed the squeaks in the floor of the apartment above me. The new tenants proved otherwise. My manager said, "Give me one day's notice and leave for two days. We'll get it taken care of." I chose to jump on it early in chemo. I didn't know what was down the road, and the squeaks were driving me nuts. Too bad I wasn't a squirrel.

§

My mom picked me up and took me to her place for a few days. On the way, we stopped at a store we'd kept taking off the "to do" list due to my feeling lousy. The Brighter Side is a boutique specializing in items for women with cancer. We looked at warm hats. News to me: Head will get cold without hair! I had a meltdown while trying on hats. I love pretty hats, not functional ones. Warm hats are definitely functional (think knitted cap). The style of all the knitted hats was the same. My hang-up became between color and yarn type. Everyone in the store pitched in:

"Oh, that's soooo perky!"

"Cute!"

"It brings the blue out in your eyes . . . ."

Chapter 9

I'd respond, "Yes, but does it look good on me?"

Then the other hat got responses of "What a beautiful color!" "That brings color to your face . . . ."

And my response, "Yes, but does this hat look better on me, or the other one?" It came down to one hat being perky, and one hat being a beautiful color. I felt I couldn't do "perky" quite yet.

Then, in less than ten seconds, I decided to get an additional hat, and everyone approved unanimously that the blue hat was for warmth, and the white hat was for my soul. I loved it! It was a broad rim, white linen hat with a leopard-print scarf wrapped around the crown.

Mom gifted me the warm "functional" hat; I bought the pretty one, and a cotton wig cap meant to wear under a wig, but I wore it at bedtime to keep my head warm. On the way out, the woman who'd worked with us asked us to wait a second. She picked out and gave me a Beanie Baby polar bear (which happens to be a strong animal totem of mine) wearing a pink T-shirt: Don't Just Survive, THRIVE!

I was worn out, and the ride to Mom's was rough. Stop and go traffic for an hour and a half. I didn't do well in the car in those days. Even with anti-nausea medication the ride had me on edge all the way. After a few days at Mom's, she brought me back to my place. Weary, I walked straight to my bed, leaving Mom in my dust, unloading her car. I woke up and had a meltdown over having too many paper towels in my 600 square foot, virtually no storage space apartment! It was ridiculous. I felt out of control over who was doing what and how in the name of helping me. The meltdown wasn't pretty, and I hoped in the future they'd be few and far between. I'd been warned chemo would play a part in my emotions while I was being bombarded with drugs and taken into early menopause. Geez!

I woke up the next morning feeling great. A much welcome feeling from the day before's implosions.

§

Three days before my second chemo, the hair on my head hurt when I woke up. It felt like it was "bent" the wrong way. They told me this would be the sign of hair loss. OH NO. It's happened. I checked. No. It isn't on my pillow, and it's still on my head, so it must be safe to look in the mirror. My hair felt brittle and was actually getting curlier. A curl near my eye changed directions, poking me in the eye instead of curling outward!

Not everyone loses all their hair with chemo. Those who don't get mighty thinned out. When the reconstructive surgeon at my consultation appointment mentioned hair loss, I immediately had a memory of being age five or six wearing a wig of my mom's. I think every woman had a wig for fun in the 1960s. This one was strawberry blonde, and hit me mid-back. With that wig, Avon sample lipstick, and Mom's high heels, I was a diva!

At that appointment, my mom also had an instantaneous memory: My dressing as a gypsy (again about age five or six), sporting a scarf on my head, eye shadow, lipstick, and jewelry — lots of it. Thank God I had the foundation of a love for hats and scarves! It would be a matter of color, style, makeup and jewelry. Attitude would take care of the rest. Hmmm . . . . I've been told I have an attitude! Let's just hope it's a positive one!

My eyebrows itched. I found myself bargaining with God: "If I can just keep my eyebrows . . . . " I caught myself a few times with this crazy phrase, and each time I'd remind myself not only does God not "do deals" but what the heck am I doing, going for eyebrows, and not a campaign to save my breast! Funny how we react in immediate fear, isn't it?

§

Walking 300 yards to Vons grocery store was big stuff for me. More of a physical and social exercise than anything else, but I felt I

Chapter 9

came home with a prize—never mind the exhaustion, and not budging an inch on the couch for an hour after.

§

There's a chant I've heard at Maundy Thursday services, "Stay with me, remain with me. Watch and pray." It's taken from Matthew 26:36-38 when Jesus is telling his disciples to sit and pray, then wait and watch. This chant penetrated me so deeply this year. The night of chemo, and the following day I felt so comforted and blessed to have had people stay with me. They prepared food—tepid chicken broth, crackers, etc. Some read to me, some held the consciousness of Light while I slept. I felt safe.

Three months before I started chemo my hair stylist moved to Texas. My stylist before that left me for Kansas! When my hair began falling out, I made an appointment to have my head shaved with Becky, my mom's hair stylist, who'd gone through breast cancer and has a memory of what a big deal the initial hair loss is.

My pattern of doing as much as I possibly could the day before chemo was in full swing. I cleaned the tub, and almost washed laundry. The door to the laundry room had already become too heavy for me. My sister came to the rescue on her way home from work. I cooked some chicken on the barbecue for lunch, handing her the spatula when I felt a wave of fatigue. She looked at it, then at me. "Turn the chicken. I'm tired." This was my first realization that people wouldn't read my mind, and they might not understand the easiest of activities would wring me out. After lunch she left. I fell asleep on the couch for an hour. (I'm seeing the benefits of couch ownership! For two years I lived without one. Never saw the need. Never had the desire. Now it's on my gratitude list.)

At my oncology appointment one day I asked, "What could've caused the cancer? How long do you think it's been in my body?"

My oncologist said the best thing I could do was to move on from questions like that. "We just don't know." That gave me a lot of peace. When I find myself digging up how, when and why, I get back on track hearing the echo, "It's best to move forward from here."

E-mail Updates
To: Bcc
Date: June 18

Here are the last two weeks:

Great news! The port has adjusted to my body, and they're now fast friends! What a joy to laugh, breathe, talk, bend and move! It makes other issues doable. I've had a fantastic week with energy, no nausea. Things seem like they're coming together.

My sleep pattern is changing. I used to stay awake from 3-6 a.m., now it's midnight to 1 a.m.. I get out of bed and practice what I'm learning on YouTube: Tying scarves, and turbans. Having my arms over my head makes me tired enough to go back to sleep. (And I'm getting pretty good with my new accessory!)

Medical folks tell me they are thrilled to have a patient with a high health base line. (Sounds funny, doesn't it? "You're really healthy—and you have cancer.") Chemo is doing its thing, moving me into early menopause: Last week I had my last period—and first hot flash.

Yesterday I met my new oncologist. I really need to walk in the room and see/feel a strong presence who can talk me off the ledge on those type of days. Someone to say, "I know it sucks—and you CAN do this." We got along fine. He has more of a "medical" attitude, sticking strictly to the facts, Ma'am. But I already feel I'm

Chapter 9

getting more answers to the questions I ask, and we both laughed a few times. I'm very happy I made the switch!

My hair has lost its volume, and is brittle.

My friend Rev. John came up from San Diego and took me to chemo #2.

That's the scoop for now.

Love you.

Peace,

C

Tips for Him or Her:

✔ Sometimes you can plan too far in advance. I was so set on planning ahead and being self-sufficient during chemo. I deep cleaned my apartment, and stocked up on food—especially canned. Keep in mind your tastes will change. I bought a double pack of spinach and cheese ravioli at Costco and put it in the refrigerator. My friend Mary, who stayed with me the night after my first chemo, saw the package and looked at the date. It had already expired! Plan ahead the best you can, then trust people won't let you starve.

✔ Keep a constant amount of a little bit of food in your stomach to decrease nausea.

✔ Avoid lying down right after eating to prevent nausea.

✔ Microwave rather than use the stove or oven to minimize food aroma.

✔ Eat food at room temperature to decrease the possibility of food related nausea.

✔ Blend: 1-2 whole leaves of chard, half a banana, and some water. It tastes better than it sounds—or looks. If you're constipated, don't knock it.

✔ Eat every one to two hours. Drink well before, or after eating. Otherwise, you'll be full, bloated, nauseous, and not eating.

✔ It's a tough balance—drinking for much needed hydration, and eating for energy, calories and protein. You may feel all you do is eat, sleep, and stave off nausea. Chances are that's all you are doing. It's your job right now. It'll get better.

✔ Contact Good Wishes: www.franceluxe.com. Their silk head wrap (for women) was incredibly soothing for the first few days after my head was shaved. Then I wore scarves.

Chapter 9

✔ Take naps. Just go with the flow. Buy eyebrow stencils, or take a close-up photo of your face before chemo begins. When you lose your eyebrows and decide to "paint them on" you'll know where they go! When they do grow back, they come in fast. It's amazing how the eyebrows frame the face.

✔ Ask those offering help to check in again down the road. Even if it's once a month, by phone, e-mail, video chat, or greeting card. When people asked, "What can I do?" I had no idea what to expect. It was too early for me to answer the question. I wanted to keep my independence and live on my own, but knew I'd need help. My not giving ideas to people gave them the impression I had things under control, or didn't want help.

✔ Get a satin pillowcase to ease the tugging on hair when it's fragile. The satin feels a bit of a luxury at a time when they are far and few. I got a great price on www.overstock.com. They come in packs of two. Gift one, keep one!

✔ Realize now: No one will do the dishes like you, clean the house like you, or drive like you. Everyone's doing their best out of love—and out of service for you. Allow them. Unless they're doing something to endanger you, give up the power struggle now. You'll experience different levels of car comfort, styles of driving, and food brand you like and don't. A lot of this is trial and error. People do things differently, and it'll serve you well to roll with as much as you can.

Tips for Those Who Want to Help:

✔ "If you need anything, let me know." It's said with good intention but can also be a cop-out. Remember a time when you've had the flu. When you've been on your knees with nausea, fever, aches, and extreme weakness. Or medicated and moving in slow motion—not able to read, let alone look up a phone number. Can you imagine in that moment being able to pick up the phone to say,

"Could you please take out my trash, or cook me a meal, or come by and let me say the word 'cancer' and cry without you getting weird about it?" By saying, "Let me know if you need anything" the ball is back in the court of the person needing help. Give concrete ideas of what you're willing to do: "I'll drop you off, pick you up, but won't wait with you." Or, "I'll deliver a meal once a week." After questioning people who offered me "anything," I learned three people didn't drive beyond a ten-mile radius of our city, and even more didn't cook.

✔ Smells/aromas can set off nausea. If you're visiting them, go easy on the perfume or cologne. Be cautious gifting flowers or scented candles.

Chapter 10

CH-CH-CH-CHIA!

AFTER CHEMO #2 (WEEKS THREE AND FOUR)

Flavors seemed to get stronger. The first bite of anything was FANTASTIC! I asked about this—I kept hearing taste would fade. My oncologist said the steroids I was taking for the first few days of each chemo round stimulated appetite.

My preference for food texture began changing at this stage. Salty, dry textures of crackers and popcorn gave way to softer foods.

Iceberg lettuce (which I hadn't had in years)—I craved it especially at 3 a.m., along with Otter Pops, cottage cheese, nectarines, apples, canned peaches and pears. I couldn't stand the texture of fresh or frozen green beans, but craved canned green beans—and, they were eaten from the can, refrigerating what was left. Mashed potato, scrambled egg. Activa yogurt. Canned chicken with only Miracle Whip. No seasoning, celery, etc. A few spoonfuls made a great breakfast, or snack. Gatorade, (flat) 7-Up, water, almond milk.

§

Mary stayed two nights after my second chemo. In the morning I asked her not to leave until I'd taken a shower. I knew hair would come out, I just didn't know how much. In the shower my hair was coming out in wads. I decided, I better just go ahead and wash it to see where this was going. It was an unstoppable mess. I didn't cry, but I did shake a lot. It helped me to know this was a sign that chemo was working, and the hair loss was medication induced, not my body just dropping hair. I've got beautiful hats, wraps and turbans—and my hair will grow back. I figure on my birthday (December) I'll have baby hair sprouting up! I see my upcoming head shave as winning the game versus being taken down one day at a time. However, having mentioned this, I feel I'll experience some resemblance to the famous Edvard Munch painting, "The Scream." I'd never once in my life bad-mouthed my hair texture, color, thickness, wave, etc. (Okay, I had a few bad haircuts.) I'd been aware how fortunate I was to have the hair I did. A year before my diagnosis, I'd grown out my hair to donate ten inches to Locks of Love because I knew it was a beautiful, meaningful gift. How ironic. Now I really understood.

§

Awful! For four days after my second chemo appointment, I'd move from the couch to the chair to the refrigerator, and back to the couch. I ached everywhere. It resembled the worst flu ever. My lips quivered—an omen that's always gotten my full attention!

I'd wake up in the middle of the night roasting hot. I'd get out of bed and have an Otter Pop (one ounce of flavored ice), then I'd have a craving for iceberg lettuce with a tiny bit of honey mustard dressing, and a few sips of 7-Up or water. Then I'd take an anti-nausea pill. This culinary delight was enjoyed with some classical

Chapter 10

music on the radio. Within an hour, exhausted, I'd toddle back to bed.

Carpet shampooer in tow, my mom and sister were at my doorstep. I perched on the couch and watched them move ninety-five percent of my stuff off the carpet. My sister got goin'—vacuuming and shampooing my apartment. It was beautiful! Worn out—them from working, me from chemo, stress, and watching them work—we all headed to Mom's, before I'd get my last hair cut for a long time.

The initial loss of hair taunted me. With every move I made, hair would fall out. I'd feel a strand of hair on my arm, my neck, down my shirt—a constant reminder of unknown things to come. I wore a turban for one day to keep the shedding to a minimum, but my head hurt from my hair being constricted. At night I took the turban off. I awoke to a pillow full of stray hair. Gross. Tape picks up only so much. The hair seemed to be everywhere except staying on my head. By making the appointment to have my head shaved, I felt I took the tiger by its tail. I was in charge—not cancer, not chemo.

I asked my mom to take pictures of the haircut. I didn't know what I'd do with them afterward, but I knew this haircut was a one-time event. I was Becky's last client of the day. My mom, Becky and I were the only ones in the salon.

Before going in, I was a wreck. I was stressed out, amped up, and scared stiff. Upon spying the empty, mint-green rigidly square barber chair, I mused, how appropriate: the electric chair. Settling into the chair, I took in a deep breath—and out came tears. Then Becky cried, and gave me a big hug saying, "I wish I could say something."

"I'm glad you aren't" (as in giving me advice, telling me it'll grow back, or it'll be okay . . .). We pulled it together, and that was the last day I cried over losing my hair.

Because my hair was so thick, Becky used sheers to give me a short haircut before shaving my head. Looking in the mirror, I admired the new style, Oh, okay, that's cute—then realized the real job had just begun. And with that, so did real ruminations. At one point, The "Mama-razzi" requested a smile.

Becky had to stop shaving several times to unclog her razor, and give my tender scalp temporary reprieve. We decided to call it quits with the "Sluggo" look. We figured in a week the stubble would either fall out, or my scalp would be less tender, ready for another shave. After washing my "hair" Becky dried my head with a towel. I howled in pain! She'd brushed velvet the wrong way.

I donned the soothing, warm silk head wrap gifted from Good Wishes. Becky put me on notice: "Complete strangers will either tell you their story, or ask about yours." I'm not thrilled about this. Not at all.

The next day: A new day! I awoke extremely pleased "the deed" was done. No hair on my pillow, falling onto the couch, the floor, or down my shirt. What a great feeling! One less worry—not to mention that of wondering whether I'd have a good looking bald head! Thank God I did. I even considered donning plenty of sunscreen and sporting my Telly Savalas head!

§

Mom and I visited the American Cancer Society, meeting a woman who'd been helpful to me on the phone. She invited me to come in and look at wigs and bangs, and said she'd teach me how to tie a T-shirt turban. While we were in the lobby, a new volunteer with a big heart (and a little thinking cap) waited for her supervisor. She kept looking over at me then asked, "Have you heard about hydrogen peroxide?"

Having no clue where this conversation was headed. I responded, "Yes."

Then she said, "Look it up on the Internet. It's supposed to be good in preventing and curing cancer."

Chapter 10

"Oh. I'm not interested in getting my medical information from the Internet." She kept insisting I check it out. I insisted otherwise. "I'm working with a medical team. I have a healthy lifestyle and habits. I'm just not interested." So, she did what any caring person would do when talking to a moron who isn't taking advice given: She asked my mom if she'd heard of hydrogen peroxide! "HA!" I laughed out loud.

She gave me one more try, saying, "Really, you should look it up—"

As she was called into a meeting by her supervisor, I remembered a note I used to have posted on my car dashboard: Never argue with an idiot. People watching may not be able to tell the difference.

In the end, only a few people shared off the wall things:

"Was it a shock when you were diagnosed?"

"It would make you pull your hair out! Well, not you. You don't have any hair." That one came from someone with a developmental disability. It actually made me laugh. I had to agree! The more common situation was people not knowing what to say. I noticed kids and the elderly were never freaked out.

E-mail Updates

> *Dear Michele,*
>
> *Man, you are so good at dealing with thinking-impaired people. I'd love some advice. Any ideas on a graceful way to honor my energy, respect kind (strange) people, and get out of the conversation?*
>
> *xo,*
>
> *C*
>
> §
>
> *hey girly . . . .*

ah yes

well several things come to mind

first

god bless your beautiful head

i know how sad and just crazy it feels

second . . . a long time ago i read or someone told me a scripture line jesus said be kind to the feeble minded and that is the bottom line we are weak/and/or feeble in our humanity

and i think when people see someone who "looks" as if they are weak, they feel the opportunity to "empower" them from their feebleness

if you can . . . just say thanks, roll your eyes and move on and realize they probably do mean well . . . it is exasperating and intrusive . . . they try to make themselves feel better by "helping" you.

say thanks, but i've got all the true support i need

of course my flippant side might start to say stuff . . .

"i'm in the telly savalas fan club, got a tootsie pop sucker"

"sinead o'connor is the leader of my band, got any requests"

"i learned everything from howie mandel, deal or no deal"

most of all keep that peace inside yourself, and when it is hard to find, get fucking mad, release the negativity around you and it will be all good again

snoopy says so

Chapter 10

big love and hugs hi fancy nancy BIG HUGS,

Michele

I kept postponing lunch with my friend Cathy because I didn't feel well. One day it finally happened. She arrived with our lunch and a big bouquet of sunflowers over two feet tall. What a lovely sight! My attention was taken off their beauty, and I spiraled into dread at the thought of getting out the proper vase. Cathy was eager to get the vase, but sometimes it takes less energy to do something than it does to give directions.

"No, behind that. Under the bottle. Yes. In the box. No. The other box . . . . " I got on the floor. (Super nauseous, and weak to boot, this was way out of my plan.) The vase I needed was in the floor level cabinet, way in the back, in a box, under things. As soon as I retrieved the vase Cathy whooshed it away to add water.

She headed for the sink. "No! Use a bucket." (There's no way the vase will fit in the sink for water, and I didn't want water spraying everywhere, or a broken vase.)

"Where's the bucket?"

Still on the floor, turning 180 degrees, pointing to the cabinet below the sink, trying to conserve my energy using American Sign Language, "Under." (Far more helpful if the recipient knows the language!). Okay, charades aren't working, get vocal.

"Your bucket is under the sink?"

Exasperated, I said, "Yes." I got off the floor and slumped onto the couch. She aimed the bucket of water over the eighteen-inch tall vase. Water poured onto the counter, to which she immediately tended, but it wore me down further.

Thinking had become a chore. So many daily changes. As Cathy prepared lunch, offering this or that, I felt bad—shooting down every idea. "Just a little—" She heaped my plate. The sight and smell of so much food was overwhelming. People didn't "get it."

I kept telling them, "My tastes are that of a four-year old. My toleration for grown up food is gone." I had good energy between 11 a.m. to 2 p.m.. Cathy arrived close to noon.

At 2 p.m. she was drying dishes. "Where does this go? Where are your empty containers? I thought you recycled."

She thought I was resting because I lay on the couch, but I couldn't fall asleep with someone asking me questions. I was wasting energy thinking for her to pick up telepathically: *Look around. Open cabinets. Notice I'm different now. I've been dragged by a truck! Stop!* At 2:10 p.m., absolutely knackered, I expelled, "Cathy, You have to leave now! Leave everything where it is." She picked up her things and left. She looked hurt. I felt bad—but was sound asleep by the time she got to her car, and I slept for two hours. People weren't factually seeing how I was. When I'd say I was having a good day, they'd think "normal" day.

I didn't know sunflowers had a smell! I was overcome with nausea when in the front half of my apartment. The flowers were beautiful. They came with love. They had to go. I gave them to my apartment manager.

§

Between my second and third chemo, I was driven to my computer session at the Apple store. (It ended up being the only one I did for six months.) I warned my drivers I wasn't chatty these days, but I think I surprised them getting in the car, closing my eyes and not saying but a peep. My driver carried my laptop for me. We walked halfway from the car to the store, then sat on a bench for a few minutes before continuing.

Sitting there, I really noticed my surroundings: The filtered sun through the blooming Jacaranda tree. Music piped through the shopping mall speakers—the song kept repeating, "What a beautiful day." Indeed. What spoke loudest to me were the "stories" of people passing by. I noticed three individuals either

Chapter 10

with a walker or limping. I presumed these people had lifelong disabilities (stroke, polio, etc.) Wow. Thank God, girl. Yours is over in a year. Your hair will grow back, reconstruction surgery will take care of your physical appearance, and cancer will be removed. Thank God. I then noticed my thinking and was pleased. It truly was a beautiful day!

Stuff only someone going through this wants (sort of) to know:

The not-so-public hair—I lost them all. Some call it "Brazilian." It's actually more of a "plucked chicken" look. My nose hair even fell out! Strange feeling, and a reminder how we take things for granted. My eyebrows thinned tremendously. I completely lost my eyelashes. Just when you think you've found a ray of sunshine in the whole hair loss thing, they tell you your leg and underarm hair will not fall out. (But it does grow very slowly.) I never knew so much was involved in having cancer. I thought, "They go bald. They get tired." That "tired" part is ridiculous! Already my immune system had dropped. My throat hurt like crazy. The big activity for me was walking to the Vons grocery store at 6:30 a.m.. The early hour shopping ensured no waiting in line, fitting into my level of stamina. It must've looked like I was in a hurry—speed walking to the one item already in mind, then to the cashier. I used a debit card for all transactions. It cut down on germs, time, and thinking.

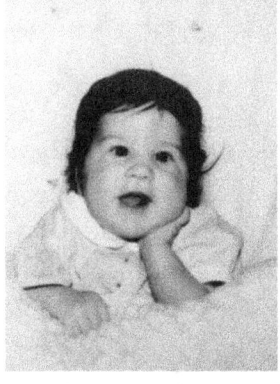

6 months with hair

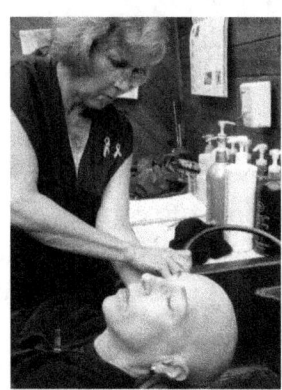

Age 44 without

My scalp was tender and itchy for two days. I used a baking soda paste the night I came home from having my hair shaved off. I found it extremely soothing. My sister prepared the paste and applied it. We laughed, as neither of us can remotely pass as Susie Homemaker, and once the paste was made, we weren't sure how to get it on my head (our mixture was runny). We were at my mom's house and Mom, who can solve any problem, was gone. We decided to pull a kitchen chair to the counter, and have me hang my baldness over the sink. My sister put the (way too goopy) mix on my head. Mom came home mid-project, and wasn't sure the situation was under control. We weren't very convincing with wide eyes and giggles.

I returned to my apartment after the few days at Mom's. The noise from the floor upstairs had been addressed. I had the front door of my apartment open while I washed dishes. I heard, "Uhh-oooh." I turned to see my next-door neighbor, a retired Marine Sergeant, fumbling for his keys to hurry inside his place. Normally, we'd exchange greetings. I realized he'd just seen me. Without warning. Without my big head of hair. From then on, my door wasn't open as often as it had been before, because I was usually lying on the couch. When we did see each other, he'd keep his conversation to "Hi." No questions. No comments. When my hair grew back, it was as if nothing happened. He'd greet me by asking how I was doing.

§

I joined a "How to Cope" conference call and was asked "What are you doing to cope?"

"I have a Wall of Gratitude—I write names, events, and things for which I'm grateful each day on shelf paper with colorful felt-tip markers. It covers my living room wall, like wallpaper." Everyone on the call (eight of them) shared how it took a newcomer to the group to point out something so uplifting, yet so easy. Reading the

Chapter 10

ongoing list of good in my life lifted me, and thrilled those who came to visit me. They'd share their favorites, and were genuinely touched seeing their name on the list. I kept the list going May through October. It was even filmed by a local TV news crew.

E-mail Updates
To: Bcc
Date: June 27

> *Here are some photos of the big event from the past two weeks. I've got a good-looking baldhead! Thank God!! (Believe me, you start to worry about this sort of stuff!)*
>
> *This week I had one really bad day—off the charts. Followed by a rough day, but at least on the radar. Then a really good day. My need for anti-nausea meds has been less on the overall need, and more when I do need them.*
>
> *I'm livin' the life of a cat: Eat a little, sleep a little, stretch a little. Repeat.*
>
> *Thanks for all your love and support. Have a FANTASTIC day!*
>
> *Love, Claudia*

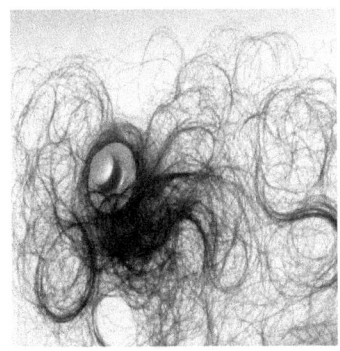

After second chemo

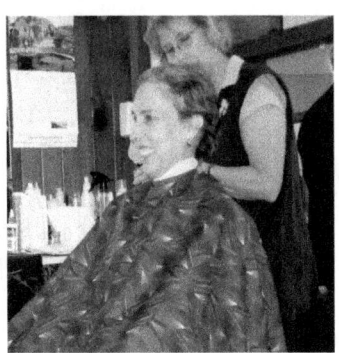

Oh, OK, that's cute . . .

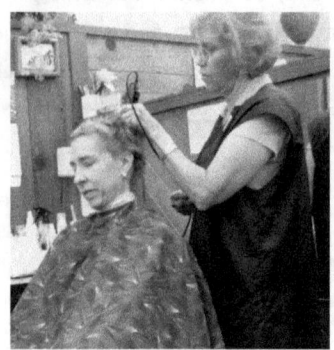
I'm really going to be without hair

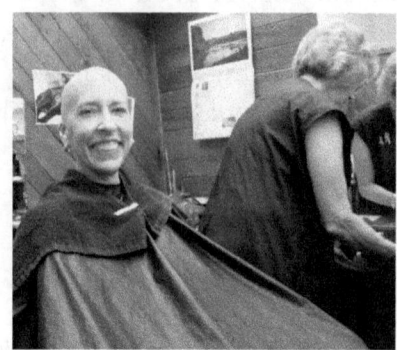
Feeling like I took the tiger by its tail

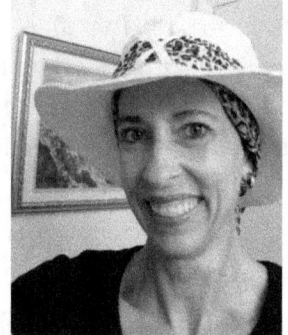
Have makeup and accessories, will smile

Happy with the outcome.

§

What's up Sweetz?!

It was really nice to speak with you last night. I felt proud of myself for not talking on and on for thirty minutes! Yes, it's still all about me!

It hurt my heart to read your message around your hair loss . . . but I got over it as soon as I scrolled down to the

Chapter 10

pictures. For truly beautiful women, hair is just another accessory . . . and yours will be grown back in no time—along with the rest of your perfect healing! I think the shorter look becomes you! And you've gotten pretty clever with the scarves and hats! It sounds like you're more comfortable—I trust that's the case.

So I heard from the [seven day silent retreat] Vipassana folks. I can't wear shorts! What's a fella to do??? They told me the pajama type pants I have would be fine! I'm headed to Hippieville!

Well I'm gonna close for now. I'm speaking tomorrow and waiting for inspiration. You take care of yourself, ya heah?!

love,

MC

§

It's gone 11 p.m. so gotta go to bed cos exam tomorrow BUT opened your e-mail. You would fit right in on a Paris street, a very sophisticated look (OK maybe not baking soda-head one). All you need is a carry bag with a poodle in it.

Cheers for now,

Allan

Tips for Him or Her:

✔ Have dental work, including cleaning, done prior to chemo. It's highly recommended not to have dental work during the months of treatment.

✔ Keep your mouth as moist as possible during the months of chemo treatment. Dry mouth is a perfect host for bacteria, causing cavities and other dental problems. Gum moisturizes the mouth, and gives your jaw some chewing exercises.

✔ Reduce dry mouth with Biotene, or any other alcohol-free toothpaste and mouthwash. It really works! I used the mouthwash throughout the day with exception of when I had mouth sores (when the object was to keep the mouth dry). After chemo, I "wowed" my dentist with having "only" one cavity.

✔ Apply for Cleaning for a Reason: With verification from your doctor, this service provides four months of monthly, general cleaning at no charge. www.cleaningforareason.org.

✔ Discuss with your doctor whether to take vitamins during chemo. I was encouraged not to take them during chemo, clearing all obstacles from its path. Chemo's job is to kill all fast growing cells—good along with bad. Vitamins build up the body's immune system.

✔ Get a cotton wig cap before your haircut. The seams are on the outside; they're comfy and cozy for bedtime. Any wig store or cancer specialty shop will have them. Make an appointment for your hair to be shaved off, versus waking up with chunks on your pillow. My hair began to fall out two days after my second chemo. It taunted me, one hair at a time. What empowerment to shave it off before it all fell out! Some women choose to have a friend shave it off, others go to a barber. My prerequisite was that the person shaving my hair was a woman who had gone through chemo-induced hair loss.

Chapter 10

✔ Put your shaved hair in a potted plant outside for the birds building nests! That's what a friend of my mom's did after her daughter lovingly shaved her head.

Tips for Those Who Want to Help:

✔ Get a box of baking soda to soothe an itchy, achey, post-shaved head. Pretend you're making brownie mix! Pour the baking soda and lukewarm water into a big bowl, mix with a spoon for about 50 strokes. Yummm . . . . The mixture consistency should be thick enough to not run into their eyes. Spread the mixture on their head, and leave it anywhere from five minutes to an hour. Rinse off with lukewarm water. You can use this mixture as often as you want for one to three days, until itching and soreness are gone. My mom's friend said Selsun Blue soothed her tender, itchy scalp the day of her haircut. I only knew the "Chia Pet" approach—the look you'll get with baking soda.

✔ Run errands to get Biotene, a cotton wig cap, baking soda or Selsun Blue.

✔ Offer to shave their head, make the paste and apply it for them.

Chapter 11

FIELD TRIP!

AFTER CHEMO #3 (WEEKS FIVE AND SIX)

My iron level was low. If it got too low, they'd postpone chemo. It sounds nice, but it isn't "cancel" chemo—it's postpone—and I was determined this process wasn't dragging out! On my chemo weeks, I ate high iron foods, especially a few days before my blood draw to ensure my chemo stayed on schedule.

A few days before getting mouth sores, I craved corn tortilla chips. My diet seemed to be focused on iron at this stage. Cheese pizza (room temperature). Pizza is high in iron. Canned green beans (higher in iron than beets). Watermelon (high in iron). Split pea soup (high in iron). Canned pears. Avocado, corn tortillas with cheese and a tiny bit of chicken from a can. Milkshake with a few slices of banana, some pear, blueberry, or whatever the mouth and stomach can tolerate. Cottage cheese. Gatorade, (flat) 7-up, water, and just for a new flavor, super diluted cranberry juice. Every thing was leaving an aftertaste, and juice alone was too acidic.

§

I asked my oncologist, "Why haven't I ever seen people with cancer at the beach?"

"Probably because they're low on energy, and chemo makes most people photosensitive." I quickly learned "photosensitive" was code for "can't see a thing through squinting eyes even while wearing sunglasses."

§

Fourth of July weekend Mom came up to visit. I was in my two-day post-chemo fog, where I didn't do anything. Every two hours I'd sleep for two hours. I began to feel the "48 hour crud" creep down my body as Mom prepared to leave. I announced, "I feel fluffy." Realizing that wasn't the word, I stopped. "No. Puffy." Then searched again for another word.

Mom scrunched her eyebrows, "Swollen?"

"Yes." It's a trip, this journey. An absolute trip!

The pain after chemo started in my neck, then moved down the arms, body, and legs. The next day I'd be a goner. It felt like the worst flu ever. Reading was out because my vision and concentration was fuzzy. Talking took too much effort, eating wasn't satisfying and came with the possibility of not staying down. Discomfort was the norm for two days. My fantasies of being anywhere else, doing anything else, were numerous.

There were days I did nothing but lie on the couch, move to the bed, the refrigerator, and back to horizontal. Days three through five after chemo I'd feel really nauseous, and decide to either take medication to prevent the feeling but give in to deep sleep, or be awake with quaky lips and a very uneasy feeling of what was around the corner. I slept nineteen to twenty-one hours a day.

My emotions went up and down, especially on rougher days. I cried easily. I came across a photo I'd taken of four people on a bridge under which our ship was passing in Norway. One of the people on the bridge is waving to us; another is taking our photo as we're waving back—taking photos of them. Seeing this photo of

Chapter 11

kindred souls—just as thrilled to see us as we to see them—brought me to tears.

Some days, seeing couples doing laundry together, I felt alone. Not that I wanted lengthy conversation, but just to touch base with someone. Someone to pour me a drink, cut a nectarine for me. What a luxury! How fortunate I was. Mom and Mary served me as if I were the Divine.

§

Six days after my third round of chemo I woke up to mouth sores on my gums. I referenced what I've come to call "The Book of Paranoia." Actually, it's called *Chemotherapy and You*, by the National Cancer Institute. It's a very good source of information, and is well written. I looked up "mouth sores." The instructions read: Notify your doctor immediately if you notice mouth sores. Rather than having someone drive me twenty-one miles each way, my doctor called in a prescription to a nearby pharmacy. I asked my apartment manager if he'd mind going to pick up my prescription, and without hesitation he agreed. The pharmacy didn't have the full dose of mouthwash readily available, so they sent my manager away until they could talk with my doctor. (Yes, there's a mouthwash out there that requires a prescription.) A few hours later, my manager delivered a two-day dose.

"There's no charge today. Tomorrow, the pharmacy will have the remainder."

After I swished and gargled the first of my four-times-a-day doses, I began to feel nauseous—a side effect of this mouthwash! Tired of it all, I started to weep, which turned into full-on crying. I had a short chat with God. Okay, I need to have someone reach out to me. Someone who can help me. Within thirty minutes I got a call from a friend I hadn't seen or talked with in several months.

"Claudia! You've been on my mind. Is it a good time to call?"

Within minutes of hanging up with her, Mary called.

"Just checking in. How are you today?"

After a nap I checked my e-mail. I'd received a one-liner from Michele:

"You are completely supported. Big love." Attached was a picture of an angel.

Thank You God. I don't like this journey. I don't understand this journey. But I do understand that I'm loved and supported.

That night I noticed red blotches on the base of my head and neck. Great. I've got a good-looking head and now I have red blotches to contend with. I didn't know if it was from lying on it so much, or what. It was a disappointment, either way.

After a week of feeling awful, I had a good day. My mom came up. We made a list of things I needed. I pushed for a field trip.

"Let's go to Costco!"

After I shared my strategy plan, she reluctantly agreed. Mom dropped me off at the tables in front, where I sat and waited for her to park. In Costco, we dashed to the back for the water, dashed for this and that, and then I led Mom in a speed walk to the shortest checkout line. In less than thirty minutes we finished the trip, and were back home. Mom unloaded her car, making several trips with water bottles in her tote bags, as I took a thirty-minute catnap.

Next trip: The pharmacy for the remaining prescription mouthwash. I felt confident I could walk with Mom to the pharmacy, just on the other side of Vons grocery in the strip mall. I called ahead:

"Is the prescription ready? Is there a line?" The coast was clear.

We walked to the pharmacy and immediately I needed to sit down. I brought $15.00, as I figured prescription mouthwash would be more than over-the-counter stuff. The pharmacist rang it up.

"$101.59."

"HUH?!" Thank God for medical coverage! "Do I really need that much?" (Yes, I found I did.)

Stunned, I sat back down. Then, I waited. And waited. I've yet to figure out what exactly takes most pharmacists so long to fill a

Chapter 11

prescription. Mom walked back to my apartment to get her car—both of us realizing I wasn't walking home. After the 0.1 mile drive, I took another nap.

We had one more errand. Off to the store for a dish scrubber. By now, the day's activities were catching up to me. We came home, and yes, I took another nap—my third. A few hours later Mom left. That night I slept nine hours, only waking for an Otter Pop, some avocado and a spoon of yogurt, which stung the sores in my mouth.

The next day I woke up exhausted. I put the trash bag at my front door for the manager, and then collapsed onto the couch. The doorbell rang at 10 a.m.. I didn't budge. Several seconds passed. I managed to move the blanket away from my face so I could see the person walk away. My manager was peering in the window. With great effort, I vaguely moved my hand, making the "turn-the-door-knob" motion. He did. He'd come to see if I wanted him to go to the pharmacy to pick up the remaining prescription. I gave an account of our trip yesterday. We both laughed incredulously at my giving him $15.00 a few days earlier in preparation for a "prescription-priced" mouthwash. I stayed on the couch all day.

§

In August, I considered the possibility that depression had snuck in. I was spending much of the day in my head. That isn't a good place for someone with so much time—especially if not feeling well. I felt overwhelmed with uncertainty around my next step in treatment, my income, my ministry, and what would unfold with the relationship between John and me.

John had been in Afghanistan for seven months. The last e-mail I'd received from him was May 22 (five months into his six month duty). He'd just learned he was being transferred to Europe after Afghanistan. John expressed his disappointment with his next assignment being overseas, wondering how we'd move forward. I continued sending short e-mails with photos from the beach and a winter in Lapland for a moment of "burr" in Afghanistan's 115°. I made the e-mails about John, not me. When he'd get to a city with Internet access, I wanted him to know he was cared for; not forgotten or given up on. Some people told me he may have been injured or killed. I knew he was alive. I also knew he didn't like being there. I had nine photos of him around my place. Those photos anchored me. They encouraged and reassured me to keep advancing in my health.

E-mail Updates

Jenny and Judy: These sisters are cousins of mine. Wildly creative! Before cancer, we'd only seen each other about five times in our lives. When they learned I'd been diagnosed, they began e-mailing me on a regular basis. Judy made me some scarves.

> . . . . *On the other hand I know you are very strong and don't complain because you've been through so much. How are you really? Lay it on me; I can take it. You are my inspiration, my friend and my cousin!!!!*
>
> *Lots and Lots of Love,*
>
> *Jude*
>
> *p.s. Scarves are W.I.P., Work in Progress in garmento lingo.*

§

> *Dear Judy,*
>
> *Lay it on you? I'm JUST NOW coming out of the worst @#$%*! four-day flu-like feeling anyone could ever have. My body's been achey, my head's been pounding, and with every move, bite, or drink I've felt like vomiting — but the great news is I haven't! I'll do anything to avoid*

Chapter 11

that part of chemo reaction. Sleeping lots. Wake up with hot flashes. They're chemo induced. Today I spent much of the day weeping—just hurting, realizing I'm a bit depressed, and I'm not even half way through this. The fear usually hits on Sun the week of chemo. It hit today. (It's 8 days before I go back!) Man, better reframe my thoughts! What a waste to worry for an entire week!! I was warned the first four days after each treatment could be really rough. Knowing that really helps me.

There. That's the factual stuff of how I feel. I DO know this will pass. It's temporary. I'm not dying, but healing. I've got fantastic support from people around the nation (very little of it is local, but it's strong from all corners!). I feel the love, and believe me, that helps!!! I'm keeping a gratitude list on shelf paper—it's my living room wall paper. You and your family are on it. No matter how bad the day is, I can come up with something for which I'm grateful. There's a pony in this pile of poop! Stop whining. Get back to the Truth that life is good, and it's a privilege.

Thanks for being in my life.

Love in huge amounts!

C

§

Marilyn: Before my moving an hour north, she was my minister for eleven years. When I was diagnosed, she was one of the first people I turned to for spiritual support.

Dear Marilyn,

I'm sorry this isn't a cheery note. I appreciate your prayer support and am asking for it right now.

I thought I'd be spending these four months walking the beach, or reading. Those plans are nixed. I'm too sun sensitive and low in energy. My eyes tire easily and are either dry or tear most the day. My concentration stinks. I get two sentences max, so Mom calls with daily devotional readings.

The updates I send out take me one week of good days to put together.

I thought of you several times today and decided to act on it.

Thanks for your support. You are truly a mentor and friend. I love you.

Love,

Claudia

§

To: Bcc
Date: July 8

Back for the touchup shaving of my head. It didn't hurt my scalp one bit!

Know of any job openings for a sitting or napping mannequin?

About three days before chemo I begin to panic, thinking of places far, far away to travel (if I had the energy). I have a medication that shuts down the nervous system if severe vomiting begins. These same pills are for anti-anxiety, to take the night before chemo. I figured I could enter my third round of chemo without jitters the night before. Guess not. I didn't take a pill last night and now at 4 a.m. realize that's foolish. Part of FLOATING

Chapter 11

through this is TRUSTING. Giving up control of what is really out of my control. I've got the tools, so now must use them.

> *"To gain control, we must give up control."~ Buddha*

The Dr. team has suggested counseling. I may go for it. I'm between thinking it'll help and thinking it'll just focus on the issues. They say I look good and seem stable but they're picking up on stress and worry beyond medical issues. Maybe if I've got someone to dump on, I'll move through this easily and gracefully—that's my prayer. Counseling may be with a social worker, or with a psychology intern. Either way, right now I like the idea of dumping on a stranger who doesn't have an emotional tie to me.

Chemo #3 (last Wed) lasted two hours longer than usual. I felt some burning pain at the port site with the saline before the chemo. That concerned them enough to hold up before starting chemo. (If there's a burning feeling during chemo it's a signal that something could be wrong.) They didn't want what seemed a minor burn to mask a possible second, more serious burn.) They ended up taking out the catheter that gets plugged into the port, and started over. We think the new tape they used to hold things in place created a reaction/red mark on my chest after just a few minutes, and that the alcohol used to clean the site wasn't dry before injecting the needle—so alcohol got into the site. (As they cleaned the site a second time, I half jokingly blew on the site to dry it off more quickly. I got busted—"you're blowing bacteria on it!" They had to clean it a third time.) Good news is that again I had a bed in a private room. I listened to my gratitude and forgiveness meditations then got some sleep. It was a really long day: 11 a.m. to 6 p.m. at the clinic. I don't expect the days to be that long again.

I've had a rough week. I keep thinking I'm coming out of it. My skin has gone a little gray, and I woke up to mouth sores this week. (Which means I can also wake up to having them GONE!)

My concentration is laughable.

Thanks for keeping the faith. The only way through this, is THROUGH it.

Please continue to know ease and grace are my path.

I'll keep you posted in two weeks.

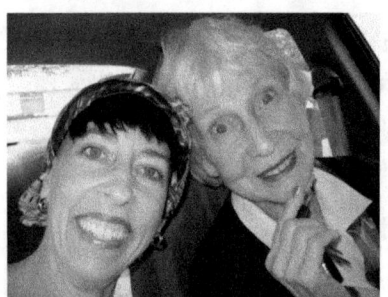
All dolled up to go home

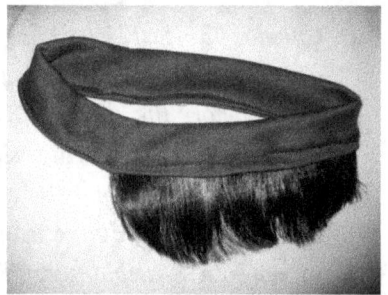
Bangs wig

As much as I liked these bangs, I only wore them this day. They were hot and I soon learned I wasn't going anywhere other than the doctor or grocery store.

Love,

Claudia

Tips for Him or Her:

✔ Keep (another) box of baking soda handy. You may still have the one from your Chia Pet days! If you ever see white spots on your gums—no matter how faint, or small—swoosh a mixture of water and baking soda around your mouth, gargle, and call your doctor immediately.

✔ Use a straw, especially if you have mouth sores. The liquids will bypass your mouth, while allowing you to keep up with hydration. The straw also aides to protect your teeth from juice stains. Remember to drink slowly, or you'll fill up on liquid.

✔ Avoid group snack platters, and salad bars. It'll help you avoid germs from those who don't wash their hands, sneeze near food, or return for more after licking their fingers.

Tips for Those Who Want to Help:

✔ Cook a meal. Bring leftovers from last night. Bring a portion to freeze, or for immediate eating. Fried or greasy food can increase nausea. If someone has mouth sores, avoid acidic or spicy foods. Their tastes and food tolerance will vary—maybe week to week. It's helpful to ask, "What sounds good this week?"

✔ Wash and put their dishes away. Clean windows, toilet, shower. Vacuum, sweep, mop. Make their bed, fluff pillows—and you get a five star rating for thinking to fluff a feather bed, if they have one! Take out the trash, replace trash bags, sanitize counters, doorknobs, etc. If you see something needing attention, do it. It doesn't have to be hard or time consuming. If you come to visit and do one chore, or fill one special request they have, you are golden!

✔ Pick up medication from the pharmacy for them.

Chapter 12

EGGS, PLEASE

Some days were compilations of depressive meltdowns. One day, within minutes of a drop-and-dash visitor, my sister arrived. We walked my ten-minute walk. As she took out my trash and left, Mary arrived to pick up her yoga DVD I never watched—let alone tried to do! Frustrated at the third week of all or nothing, I burst into tears. Two weeks prior, I wasn't even stepping out my door for fresh air. Adding to my isolation, I'd seen only two people. Last week I didn't have any visitors until Thursday, then had several in two days—proving too much activity, too close together. This week, within one hour I had three visitors!

Mary stayed while I opened a can of split pea soup. Never mind it was seventy-two degrees outside; I wanted to raise my iron levels for the upcoming blood draw in two days. Split pea soup sure tastes better when it's cold outside. Having someone with me during meals was helpful, especially if they prepared the meal. The less involvement with food preparation on my part, the more interest I had in eating. Any meal that tastes better during chemo is a big perk! When Mary left, I was worn out from the "social hour of the week" and immediately took a two hour nap. People often left when it was time to eat. I love breaking bread with others. If someone asks you to stay during their mealtime, please consider it. Or, consider coming to visit during that time.

I went through a phase getting bent out shape over people not staying during mealtime, or not eating my food. I took it personally. After all, my diet wasn't exactly enticing. I shared my view of the situation with Mary and Mom. Okay, more like I flipped out, and nearly held each hostage on separate occasions. They wanted to ensure I wouldn't run out of food—apparently thinking I offered it to anyone walking past.

The evening of my three visitors, Mom and I had an appointment to Skype each other at 7:00 p.m.. At 6:45 p.m. Dad Skyped me! This was the second time he inquired, "When are you going to wear a wig?" (Don't ask anyone this. They may not plan on the wig route.)

"If you see me wearing one, then you'll know I've decided to do so." The wig question is in the same category as handing a woman going through breast cancer a Victoria's Secret catalog or hair accessories.

My dad didn't understand why I was so upset over the question. "Your e-mail update had a photo of you with bangs." He and I kept it short. Mom and I Skyped as scheduled. A few minutes after we ended, the phone rang! I asked my friend to call another day. I'd gone from alone and depressed this morning to a deluge of visitors. It reminds me of The Metaphysician's Curse, "May all your good come at once!" (We just can't handle it.)

In the end, I never wore a wig and only once did I go bald. Even then just hanging around the apartment I wore a scarf. They were comfortable and looked good on me.

Before I lost my hair, I briefly considered a curly, ash-white wig. It was so different from the wavy, mink colored hair I've always had. The wig cost $200.00 and I wasn't sure I'd wear it much. The issue of wig care, and cautions of real versus synthetic hair played into my decision, too—I'm told when you see a woman running away from an outdoor heater, or having her husband open the oven at home, you know she's wearing a real hair wig. They

Chapter 12

catch fire very easily, and steam permanently takes away any curl or wave from them.

Days became like Jenga. What used to be easy became an effort and brought me crashing down. If I was sad, I became sadder for being so aware. I'd cry, then cry more for crying. Just when I thought I couldn't handle anything more, a big surprise arrived. I'm in the thick of chemo—with a period! I'd been advised that because of my age, I might never have a period again, especially during chemo treatments.

§

I had reached the tipping point. I had a talk with Spirit.

"Look God, if you're taking me—do it! Do it now. Do it quickly. You aren't dragging my family or friends through this! I won't allow the ups and downs of cancer to be part of my ongoing life."

Later that week I had my fourth of eight chemo treatments. My oncologist joyfully greeted me, sharing the good news: "The tumors have shrunk more than 50%." Hooray! The tumors got the message to keep shrinking—they may as well shrink down to nothing!

I optimistically asked the doctor if the shrinkage meant I'd no longer be scheduled for an October mastectomy. He was frank, telling me straight up that I was having the surgery. I sat sobbing. Like a true father of preschoolers, he asked, "Are you crying happy tears from your tumors shrinking?" He always seemed to shine the light on the areas where I'd gone dark. His question reminded me to celebrate the tumors shrinking! I smiled. Sobbing, I shook my head. "Is it about still having surgery?" I nodded. With compassion he put his hand on my shoulder and held it tight.

"There are no studies for chemo without surgery. It's just too risky." Again, he tried to help me reframe by adding, "You're halfway through the chemo part of treatment."

"Half way through means torture for another two months."

He continued to talk me off the ledge, asking if I wanted to postpone this chemo.

Mopping up my tears, I said, "No. I'm ready." I walked down the hall to my fourth chemo.

§

The meltdowns kept coming. Some days I cried all day and didn't go out at all. Mom called. She'd spoken with a woman at the American Cancer Society. They had a lengthy conversation about my sliding further into depression. The woman asked my mom to have me call ACS for a session with a counselor. Per my mom's request, I called. At 4:45 p.m. I left a message asking for a call back. (It took three weeks to find a counselor. They could do one session. It never materialized.)

A week later, after much contemplation, I e-mailed the cancer clinic's social worker, requesting help. A week passed, I hadn't heard back. Mary continued to suggest I call my oncologist to tell him I was on day ten of my period. "If he doesn't seem worried, fine, but at least tell him it's taking precious energy from you."

In the morning I called the nurse and got voice mail: "I'm out of the office for the week. Do not leave a message. If this is an emergency, call 911." Hmmmm . . . .

When I last saw the doctor, it was day three of my period. I was using three pads a day. It's now day ten of my period. I'm using six pads a day. Both Mary and Dad urged me to call the doctor—not the nurse—to let him know what was going on.

I left a message with the doctor. "It's my eleventh day of a period." I got the call back from an RN covering for the one on vacation. "The doctor wants you to come in right now for blood work." (Uh . . . what's wrong with this picture?) So, I asked someone who happened to be at my place dropping off a DVD and cutting watermelon if she had time to take me to the clinic. We left right then. The purpose was to see if I needed a blood transfusion.

Chapter 12

That evening I got a call from the covering RN saying the labs looked fine with the exception of my potassium levels seeming twice as high as normal. She believed it to be a lab error, but asked me to come back tomorrow for another blood test. We continued talking and I said, "All I do is lie on the couch and cry." She asked if I was in counseling. I flipped.

"My doctor gave me the 'assignment' to contact the social worker. It took me two weeks to build up the nerve to reach out for help. It's been an additional three weeks since I asked for help—without any response! A week after my request, thinking the social worker forgot to put an 'Out of Office' response on her e-mail, I followed-up with a hand-delivered note to her office on a day I had an appointment. The note included my phone number. No call. I've continued to spiral downward." I shared with the RN that I'd been a social worker, and we had to return all communication within twenty-four hours.

"I'm going to e-mail the social worker, asking her to call you."

I laughed.

She said, "I'm marking it 'high priority,' CC-ing myself, and asking the social worker to reply to both of us."

The following morning I changed my mind, deciding not to go in for another blood test. We knew a transfusion wasn't needed. This test was to correct a possible lab error in potassium levels and would not help me conserve energy. I have a port, and yet the day before they had used my arm to get four large tubes of blood. I just wasn't up for that on the thirteenth day of my period, midway through chemo.

I got a call from the social worker in less than ten hours after the RN shared my disappointment. The following week I began seeing a counselor—a psychology doctoral student on her third of five internships. The day she called, I'd spent the morning on my couch, crying.

"I am aware I'm loved and that this 'ick' is temporary. I'm frustrated with my lack of energy and having to rely on others so heavily. Mary lives fifteen miles east, and works. Mom lives fifty miles south. Sometimes I feel let down by others. I hear from people who say they've intended to get in touch with me, then I drop off their radar again."

§

One day an older woman in my apartment complex walked past my apartment. I saw her hesitate, turn around, and come back to knock on my door. "I'm going to the store. Do you need anything?"

I didn't, but figured if I said, "No" I'd close myself off from future offers. "Eggs. I'd love if you could get me some eggs." I gave her my debit card. As she walked off, I muttered to myself, "Great. You've just given your bank card to a complete stranger." She came back with eggs. Handing me my bank card, I had a feeling she didn't use it. Later reviewing my bank statement, my feeling was confirmed.

A few weeks later, I learned the woman who got me eggs without using my bank card, moved to her daughter's home because she couldn't afford the apartment rent. It reminded me of the Bible story, Mark 12:41-44 where the rich men gave a great deal of money, and the poor widow gave a few coins. In reality, the widow gave more because she entrusted all she had.

E-mail Updates

> *Shrinking tumors, hair growing back . . . and your period! What more could a girl want! So delighted to hear the very positive news!*
>
> *Love,*
>
> *Jenny et al.*

Chapter 12

§

From: Dad

To: Mom

Dear Nan,

I called [family] and mentioned Claudia having chemotherapy. They said they knew about Claudia's cancer but did not know if it was OK to send Claudia a card or if they should just keep quiet and not say anything. This is a typical response when dealing with Claudia as everyone feels they are walking on eggshells.

§

From: Mom
To: Dad
Cc: Claudia

Dear Bill,

I called [family] this morning and reiterated the information re: Claudia. We talked about how she is doing and what sends her off and what is working for her.

Cards are welcome but NOT "get well quick," "sorry you're sick," etc. But DO send "thinking of you" and funny cards. She cannot tolerate flowers as the fragrance makes her nauseous, and as flowers die, they are messy and when bending, nausea is not the feeling she wants.

Her appetite is not always a feeling, but she knows she has to eat something anyway, and often. Liquids are most important, as the chemo fries the system. Her mouth has sores, which are being treated with special mouthwash that leaves a lingering unpleasant aftertaste, and a side effect of nausea.

Her strength is nil. The chemo has affected her eyesight and she doesn't read more than a few sentences before it blurs and she gets a headache.

She is not wearing wigs. Too hot and uncomfortable. She has a good-looking head, wears a turban and looks "model sheik." Besides, it is what it is, and one can't hide. Think of something that demanded physical and mental effort to the point of turning your innards inside out—brutal, no escape, but you knew you had to go through it. That's how it is.

We talk daily and Skype, so she can see a person, and be seen.

Thanks for writing. Hope this helps with the understanding of Claudia's journey through this.

It's like a fracture, not a sickness.

Love,

Nan

Chapter 12

Tips for Him or Her:

✔ No matter how awful you feel, the words, "Thank You" can still roll off your lips. Realize that there are days you're no treat to be around. When someone does something for you—and at this stage they're doing plenty!—thank them.

✔ Tell your doctor if you're feeling deeper than blue, crying, feeling sad, feeling alone and sleeping entire days away—sound the alarm.

✔ Ask about your options, and ask about support groups.

✔ If you don't like one group, try another—or ask if there's a psychology intern.

✔ If you think you've fallen through the cracks, ask again, and ask someone else.

✔ Talk to the social worker.

✔ Tell your oncology nurse how you're feeling.

✔ No matter how depressed you are, get dressed. Brush your teeth and wash your face. Make your bed if you can. I wore makeup six weeks into chemo. After that, I only wore lipstick, jewelry and headscarves color-coordinated with my outfits. It's no harder than putting on grungy, mismatched clothing.

Tips for Those Who Want to Help:

✔ Bring up the subject of a support group or counseling if you notice they're depressed. Either contact an agency to get information to share with them, or ask them to ask their doctor for help. Often, a patient puts on a "good show" for the doctor by dressing up, smiling, engaging in conversation and not mentioning they're at rock bottom. It would be easy for a doctor to overlook depression.

✔ Ask if it's okay to call, knowing you may get voice mail. Don't hang up. Leave a message.

✔ Run errands. Offer them to sit shotgun in the car while you go in and shop.

✔ Drive them to the beach, or somewhere else pretty, even if they sleep the whole time. Bring a towel, bucket and anti-nausea medication, just in case.

✔ Set up a time to video chat, if you can't visit in person. It's helpful for them to see someone.

✔ Call even if you think, "I just don't want to call at the wrong time." Cell phones and land lines both have voicemail providing the caller an opportunity to leave a supportive, loving message. I found e-mail and answering the phone easy. I didn't make outgoing calls unless absolutely necessary—and even then, one night I couldn't get to the phone to call someone to take me to the emergency room. Had I gotten a call that night, I'm sure I would've found a way to the phone before they hung up!

✔ Change a light bulb, fix what needs fixing if you know how. Otherwise, water plants, mow the lawn, put up or take down holiday decorations. Do what you can. Offer.

Chapter 13

LITTLE VICTORIES

AFTER CHEMO #4 AND #5
(WEEKS SEVEN, EIGHT AND NINE, TEN)

The ordeal with the mouth sores ended. The key is knowing your body, and taking fast action to call the doctor and inform them about any spots on your gums. I returned to eating what I wanted within a month of the first mouth sore.

Again, my cravings changed. Half a sandwich: Tuna with celery and ginger. Peanut butter and jelly. Ham on white bread. Baby food (sweet potato)—and after chemo number 5, I moved up to junior baby food (lasagna). I loved summer fruit! Watermelon, nectarines, peaches, apples. Yogurt. I tried tapioca (not as good as I recalled) and doughnuts (not as good as I imagined). I enjoyed frozen meals (ravioli, or spinach soufflé), but one serving size was too much for me. Avocado, string cheese. Eggs over easy on a piece of toast (it took this long to stomach two eggs). Frozen mini pancakes. I sill ate saltine crackers and still liked mac and cheese (but not until a few days after chemo). Pudding, milkshakes and popsicles count as liquids. Take in plenty of them.

I was craving rolled tacos, so I took an anti-nausea pill and gave Mom directions to Alberto's, the closest Mexican restaurant I could think of, though I'd never been. We overshot the place and made a "U" turn. "There it is!" Mom hung a quick right—no turn signal involved and a disgruntled driver on our tail. It was rather dangerous and exciting this three mile outing for rolled tacos! At home after the first bite, I realized it was the crunch and the adventure I was after, not the taco.

During this time I lost the taste for Gatorade; in fact now I hate it. I drank 7-Up (flat), water, cranberry juice (greatly watered down), and carrot juice—but go easy, it's heavier than other juices.

I was proud of my tumors shrinking, never missing treatment, and never throwing up. These are really big victories in the world of cancer.

Then things went dark. Usually, I can turn it around. I couldn't. I had too many days to myself and just enough information to be dangerous. Two months from now I'd have a mastectomy. What would my body look like? I—Ms. Affirmation, Ms. Be Positive, Ms. Love-Your-Body-Unconditionally—was looking at another opportunity to shine. But I couldn't do it. Damn. What was this all about?

Maybe it's not about the events at all. Maybe it's how we move through them. For this phase, it was one dark cloud after another. When I'd swat off worrying thoughts about the mastectomy, I'd worry about reconstruction, (which wasn't even an option two months ago). The joints in my body hurt. A common side effect from chemo. I moved like a ninety-two-year-old. My hands and feet seared with the burning sensation of neuropathy, a condition where the nerves of the peripheral nervous system are damaged. I wondered if—and feared that—I had survived cancer to have this quality of life. There were brief moments of respite in thinking of John. Of us. Then I'd jolt into thinking of my income, and wonder how in the world I'd present workshops not having any energy. I'd hear economic news reports—the sky is falling!—and tell myself, we can't all go belly up.

Chapter 13

E-mail Updates
To: Bcc
Date: July 17

Great News! My tumors have shrunk over 50% (They told me only 10-20% of people have any shrinkage.) I had my last of the first round of chemo this past Wed. and will now begin the second round. They say my nausea will be less, and I should be able to read. Hooray!!!!!

Doctors don't seem concerned about my torso gradually being covered with brown spots (think leopard). I keep pointing the spots out—you can't miss them! My face still looks good, with some days being a bit gray. There's a mix of acne and dryness, but not bad. I'm nauseous for a week after chemo, but I haven't vomited—and let me tell you—THAT is victory!!! I eat room temperature food to avoid any lingering aroma, follow a liquid diet for 24-48 hours after chemo, and take anti-nausea meds round the clock for the first week. It's all paying off.

Some days I walk up to 12 minutes, then come back and sleep one to two hours. The shot I get for my immune system causes pain in the long bones of my body, but that comes and goes. I haven't been sick, not even once! I've been vigilant about not shaking hands. I'm using antibacterial gel anytime I go out, have paper "guest towels" in the restroom. A few days before my blood draw I make sure I'm eating things high in iron because I'm determined to get through chemo without any sessions being postponed.

More Good News: Mouth sores are going away!

Love, Claudia

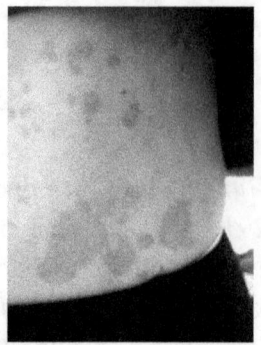

Maybe I've been wearing the Leopard scarf too much??

§

Cathy (cd): A client who became a friend. She's perky, energetic and celebrates life with flair. Her cards cheered me on.

> cd,
>
> *I'm up for a short time—these are the down days . . . .*
>
> *Lunch—Please no shellfish. Not allowed during chemo.*
>
> *I really, really do mean kid diet (bland). If you aren't up for it, fine, but I must stick to what works for me now. Today I had watermelon and a tiny bit of mac and cheese. Maybe we can get together without food? Visit will be short one, my dear—just don't have much in me now.*
>
> *I love my shirt, thank you.*

§

> cd,
>
> *I'm having a rough go here—could we pls postpone lunch? Xo C*

Chapter 13

§

Just a quick note to keep in touch. You are doing so well with this non-sickness of yours. Incredible! Hope you can hang on to the good day and keep in mind that there'll be more and more of these as time goes on.

Be in touch again soon.

Cheers for now,

Allan

§

Dear Marilyn,

I'm off to chemo now, but would like to ask for help. I've had a real hard time these past weeks. Going to a counselor tomorrow. Am on day 16 of a period, and fed up with chemo. Would you please know grace and ease for me? I know you have been, but I feel anything but that is going on now. I'm in tears all day and sleep like a champ!

I try to focus on what is working, and all the good coming out of this, but the worry seems to trump it lately.

Good news is they say I should be able to read with the new chemo I begin today.

Thanks. I really appreciate how you "get it."

xo

Love,

Claudia

§

As I hold you in the Light, I know and please know with me that you are anchored in the Light for Highest Good and complete Healing. The Universe knows only that you are in the Creative Process for complete healing and it has to respond to our direction. It is its nature to respond. So know with me that no matter what is happening in your manifest world right now, in the unseen you are moving into perfect health. Let's know that this process is moving into completion with ease and grace. I'm holding this energy of ease and grace for you. Hold this energy with me. It is your Truth.

Love and Blessings,

Marilyn

Tips for Him or Her:

✔ Celebrate victories! Did you get to the mailbox today? Did you have a visitor? A celebration might be in the form of listening to the birds outside, or sharing good news with someone—even a stranger.

✔ Take an intentional nap, soaking up the rays of the sun in celebration for a "good" day, a tumor shrinking, getting halfway through chemo—being alive.

✔ Thank your body! Give gratitude for what was, is and will be. However and whatever you celebrate, it's good for self-esteem, and your cells really enjoy acknowledgement during this love fest! Praise your body!

Tips for Those Who Want to Help:

✔ Time spent with me, and chores done for me were supreme!

✔ Give them a gift card and the field trip to use it (car wash, gasoline, grocery . . . .)

✔ Give them honest compliments. I hadn't seen my mom in two weeks. When she came up to visit, she immediately said, "Your makeup looks nice." Lying on the couch, I smiled widely. "I don't have makeup on. It's my eyebrows. They're coming back!" She noticed something changed for the better. It made me feel great.

✔ Offer to help with laundry. Load and unload the washer and dryer. Fold and put the laundry away. If they live in an apartment, gift them with a roll of quarters.

Chapter 14

DISAPPOINTMENTS

Even girlfriends flinch. Relatively new to my diagnosis, I shared the news with a friend who's a life coach. To my shock, I could visibly see her energy pull in, like a carpet rolling up. A few weeks later she called while multitasking as she drove to meet someone. Our society gives accolades for multitasking, but spirit and connections of the heart require us to be present. "How are you doing?"

"Overwhelmed. I'm doing the best I can."

"Hmmm, it sounds like you are processing."

To which I answered, "I guess that's what people do at this stage." The call immediately ceased. A year later I received an e-mail from her: *I've thought of you several times over the last few months and am finally sitting down to write a note and say hello . . . .*

Another girlfriend made the news of my diagnosis all about her uncomfortableness with the word "cancer" and her not knowing what to do. In an e-mail, she asked if I wanted a phone call. I wrote back, I need a laugh, let's talk. I signed off, FYI, I'm also uncomfortable with the term cancer being associated with me. She called, and for twenty minutes she talked nonstop about this-and-that pettiness, including dumping guys she was dating. (This stung my heart. It didn't sound like my friend, and the man I adored had recently left for Afghanistan.) This wasn't a conversation. I was being retched upon from her nervousness.

I stared at the second hand on the clock, each tick cumulative in weight. I couldn't listen any longer.

"I need to go now. I think it'll be a while before we reconnect." We hung up.

§

This isn't your time to comfort others, which is why you need to be wise with whom you share. Remember, no matter how soon after diagnosis you reveal your news with someone, you've had more time to process than they've had.

§

People, especially my family, tell me, "Others are often afraid of making the wrong move around you." I don't think the situation's that tough. If you don't know what to say, either button your lips shut—or, ask the patient (or their family) how you can help.

§

Strong men can buckle. Two men close to me reacted in ways that surprised me. These guys have heart—but coped by making jokes. That's a bad plan if the person on the other side isn't doing the same. One made a breast joke when he heard I'd had a biopsy. Never mind it was an extremely painful, completely horrible experience. The other, upon my sharing the diagnosis, carried on about getting "C" cup implants as if it had been on my wish list.

I blasted him, "This isn't about your sexual fantasy. This is about an amputation off my body!" I told him not to call me again. He wasn't currently capable of discerning appropriate comments from friendship-wrecking ones. We began e-mailing after two

Chapter 14

months. He'd signed up for a ten day, total-silence retreat and was worried about it. I was amazed he was doing it, and proud when he completed it! He first called other people when he got back—knowing he might be a loose cannon after not talking for ten days. He learned that jokes about cancer, mastectomies, reconstruction or breasts aren't in his best interest. He came down from Los Angeles twice to stay with me, once during chemo, and once after surgery. From his actions and effort, I more fully understood why he lived in a place known as "Angel City." Our friendship deepened because we both took my experience of cancer as an opportunity to grow. He later shared with me that on one of his toughest days at the retreat, he pulled out a devotional magazine. It fell open to a page titled, *I Claim Health,* by Rev. Claudia Mulcahy. He has since been called upon by others newly diagnosed with cancer, and has been of help to them.

§

During the unfolding of my diagnosis, a minister with whom I worked responded to my fear of misdiagnosis with the words, "It's all good. It's all God."

Yes, in the Absolute, it is all-good and is all God, but telling someone that in the moment they're dealing with the facts (or in my case, not dealing with them) is spiritually irresponsible.

She asked, "What would happen if it ended up being cancer?"

"They'd have to scrape me off the ceiling."

She waved her hand in the air, wiping that comment away. "You won't need that. The church will be here for anything you need. Besides, my neighbor moved through cancer just fine and I know someone's daughter who worked while going through chemo."

I know this individual meant well. I needed a different approach. We are whole, perfect and complete. Strength and faith are not about denying the condition or situation, but rather denying that the condition or situation has any power.

When a child is afraid of the dark, we (I hope) don't brush over their fear with, "The kid down the street did just fine." We show the scared child the light. We hold them if they cry. We let them be who they are. Then, we can tell them how that kid down the street was scared too, and was loved, supported, and brave—and got through it.

§

My first week into chemo, my Mom was visiting when another minister arrived with the huge Sunday flower arrangement after church. I sat and watched as the flowers got plopped onto the kitchen counter, taking up the entire space. My mom suggested I receive three flowers from the arrangement so I could enjoy the thought behind it while still having counter space.

The polite tussle of "Please keep them," "Please take them," went on until my mom said, "She can't lift it. She can't tolerate the smell, and when they fade, someone who's nauseous doesn't want to bend down to pick up fallen flowers."

A few weeks later on a Sunday the same minister called me while driving and announced, "I'm on my way over, since you're right around the corner." I seized the opportunity to request yogurt, lunchmeat, and lettuce. Her original mission was to drop off a recording of her sermon that day. The CD was blank. A "drop and dash" occurred. I felt as if I had the plague. Hurrying out the door, she said, "The quick delivery's to conserve your energy." She left. I put the food away. Head's up—that didn't conserve my energy. There are those who "get it," and those who don't. Those who don't are often the ones assuring you they do.

The following week, while I lay on my couch, I got another call from the "drop and dash" minister, "I'm on my way to come by."

Chapter 14

I'd gone all week without seeing anyone. I said, "It's not good timing; my sister's on her way."

She trilled, "I have a little something for you."

I lost it. Sobbing and ranting, I blasted her with a week's worth of isolation, fatigue, and disappointment. "I don't need things. I need help! My sister's on her way." Cathy would sometimes stop on her way home from work in Los Angeles. She'd gift me with walking around the block, cleaning windows, washing dishes, or vacuuming. She'd stay for ten to twenty minutes which was a perfect time frame for both of us. My visitors arrived within five minutes of each other. One "dropping off" a fancy wrapped package. I was a poor host, upset that my request for her to drop by another time, and not bring things wasn't honored.

Before this, she'd send me e-mails: "Waiting to do whatever you need." I'd reply with excitement, "Would love a twenty minute beach visit!" (Less than a mile from my place.) I got upbeat e-mails in return, reminding me, "All is well." Offers kept coming my way. None of the offers from this good-intending individual manifested into action.

§

I learned people do what comforts them. We like to think we reach out, but ultimately, we work within our own comfort zone. I felt like an item to be checked off this woman's predetermined "Things To Do" list. I sent one last e-mail: "I didn't realize how busy you are. I wish you the best. I've needed help and follow through. I'm requesting no more contact." So much was promised. I felt abandoned by my church, but I believe they believe they'd served me. It's all perspective.

Four people signed up at church to help me. What sort of staff minister had I been? To what sort of congregation did I belong? I admit, I wasn't open to "just anyone" coming by. I didn't want the "lookie-loos" to come by out of curiosity, or someone in need of counseling. That was a tough sale for some. It was hard enough to get those who really knew me to understand my new level of need. A minister friend pointed out to me, "Four people. That's 25% of the congregation, and if the church were one hundred people strong, don't think twenty-five people would rush forward."

I ended up with two helpers, one of whom was anorexic, so food help was out. She was golden for transportation. The other woman also a reliable driver, cut the occasional watermelon, and brought me DVDs from the library.

A major manifestation of help in the area of food and love came from a congregation, a denomination other than my own. My only connection to this church: My financial advisor. A reminder not to compromise on a dream or prayer, but to compromise on how it will come true.

It became clear to me I needed to leave my church. I met with a minister and returned my keys. We parted with closure and integrity. I felt an incredible lightness as I walked away.

Chapter 14

Tips for Him or Her:

✔ Know there will be those who love you, and who promise to keep in touch—and won't. Especially if you're not initiating contact. There will be those who tell you they're ready and willing anytime to do anything—but the fact is they're too busy. To some, offering help is automatic, with no follow-through. It's like asking, "How are you?" while continuing to walk past someone. Get over any hurt this causes, and find people who can support you and bolster the strength you have within.

✔ Use antibacterial gel or wipes after going in public. Keep some in your car. Use the wipes on shopping carts. Wipe down your wallet if you lay it on the store counters.

Tips for Those Who Want to Help:

✔ "Is there something you'd like to talk about?" "What are you in need of having done?" Perfect questions to ask them, or their family.

✔ Learn to be okay with silence. Some people feel they need to fill a break in conversation. They may want someone near, but not always talking. Some of the most powerful love and healing moments happen in the hush.

✔ Go to the store for them. Have follow-through. Put things away, or ask, "What can I do for five minutes to help out?" When a non-core support person would leave, I'd usually turn around to find something I wished I'd asked them to do, or wished they'd seen and done on their own. I valued service more than things given as gifts.

Chapter 15

THE COUCH

Three rounds into chemotherapy (July) I quit wearing makeup. Even applying it while sitting down took too much effort. I wasn't going anywhere, anyway. I continued to wear styles and colors that looked good on me, and coordinated scarves with my outfits. None of it took extra effort—so many think it does.

§

As a child, I loved my blue satin bed comforter. Now I spent my days lying on the couch wrapped in a green fleece blanket, washing it when I knew I could get through a few hours without it. Guests got other blankets, not this one. No way.

§

I heard some people didn't keep in touch out of concern of waking me from sleep. While I appreciate their consideration, these same people who didn't want to disturb me with a call didn't send a card or an e-mail, either. Who knows, perhaps we would've even had a short conversation. Maybe someone—even if not me—

would've answered the phone, or maybe the caller would've had the opportunity to leave me a greeting after only two rings.

People would say, "Call me." I couldn't remember numbers and didn't have the energy to look them up, or go through the motions of making a call. What's wrong with risking calling at a "bad time" and being told, "Thanks for calling. Wonderful to hear your voice. Could you call again in a few days?" If there's no answer, find another way to connect.

Daily, Mom called me. Sometimes twice. Our calls were short and I looked forward to them. We were Skyping, until she had trouble with her computer. That same month, my Dad had trouble with Skype. "The baby monitor" hadn't worked out as planned. It's not that someone with cancer becomes anti-social, but perhaps they do become less social. Their energy is very limited. Priorities get really clear. For me, it came down to wanting to talk with people with whom I had a strong foundation.

§

Switching to the second type of chemo, Taxol, was supposed to be easier on my body, but I was flat out exhausted, and my mouth sores worsened; I had excruciating bone pain, and a visit to the emergency room for what is considered a high temperature during chemo.

The rule is to call the on-call doctor and go to the emergency room if your temperature reaches 100.5. I had chemo on Wednesday. Friday night I had a fever of 100.8. I couldn't believe it. I wasn't up for an emergency room visit—mainly because I didn't know how I'd get to the hospital. At 9 p.m. I couldn't think straight. I lay on the couch, motionless. Finally, I got up for an Otter Pop. My temperature went down to 100.6. It took everything I had to look up the on-call number. Then, with that number in front of me, I didn't have any energy to dial or talk. I lay back on the couch,

Chapter 15

phone on my stomach. The fever began to wane. It dropped to 100.4, then at 5 a.m., I felt it break.

My mom came to visit the next day. I spent all day worrying—what if it happens again tonight? As Mom prepared to leave at 8:30 p.m. I freaked out. My temperature was 99.4. I feared it would continue to rise as the night progressed, and I was alone. My mom put her things down and suggested I called the on-call doctor.

The doctor called back. "This happens all the time. People don't call because they want to avoid the emergency room. But, your risk of infection is so high due to your immune system being basically nonexistent at this point in treatment. I know you don't want to, but go to the emergency room because of your having a fever last night."

When the ER nurse came to access my port, she didn't use anything to numb the site. At the clinic, I'd always been asked if I want lidocaine (and I always say yes). I've never felt the effects of such a big, square needle in my life. Half talking with herself, she mentioned, "I always forget to have it in a certain direction." As if working a Master's combination lock, she "dialed" the part she had just plugged into my port. It hurt, I never had anyone at the clinic do that. By looking at her face, I could tell she wasn't getting blood. I asked her.

She said, "No. How straaange . . . ." She had me move my arm above my head.

"I've always been told I have great blood return, and it's always on the first attempt." I asked her to get another nurse who could do this. I didn't like how things were going. She retrieved another nurse, who showed up with the lidocaine, per my request. After a shot of the local anesthetic, my port was accessed a second time. Immediately blood was retrieved. They gave me a surgical mask to wear to keep germs at bay, followed by a urine test, vitals, x-rays, and saline through an I.V. to rehydrate. Three hours later I got the okay to go home. The ER technician unhooked the outside catheter from my port, then realized it hadn't been flushed with saline to rinse the port clean. He flushed it directly, meaning another needle poked into my port. That night's visit could've all been done with one needle, but it took three.

The ER doctor came in to say goodbye. "Fever's a common side effect of Neulasta, the medication you're taking for an immune system boost. Continue to come to the ER if your temperature's over 100.5 because it could be really serious." I absolutely loved the ER doctor.

Mom and I were home just after midnight. She stayed the night. I gave her my bed and I slept on the couch—something I've gotten good at!

Around this time, I started wearing a surgical mask to go out. It prevented inhaling car exhaust, or freaking out if anyone coughed without using the "Dracula cough" (coughing into the crease of their bent arm). I even brought the mask with me when I went outside just to sit, in case flying debris sailed by in a gust of wind. I had a woman step back from me in line ordering sandwiches at the grocery store. I think she thought I had H1N1 (swine flu). I opted not to tell her that the mask or my hair loss weren't from my being "sick." I noticed two reactions when I wore the mask: Those who saw the mask and nothing else, and those who took in the whole picture. I didn't see people staring, but rather going through a story in their minds. I'm not sure if anyone could tell when I smiled while wearing the mask. I caught one woman in the checkout line next to me "going through her story." (My story about her is she's known this journey either personally or through someone she cared about.) I caught her "reading" me, and I winked at her. She gave me back a big smile. It felt like a "Go get 'em, girl!" moment.

E-mail Updates
To: Bcc
Date: Aug 2

Chapter 15

I know you've enjoyed some humor and photos in the updates—maybe in a later one. I've been working on this all day, 15 mins at a time, then back to couch for a lie down....

I've been off the radar for over a week.

Lower eyelashes are gone. Mouth sores have progressed, appetite is down, stomach hurts as lining is gone.

On my "high energy day" last week the maids I have once a month woke me up to tell me they were leaving. I thought maybe they didn't vacuum to avoid disturbing me on the couch. I then looked at the carpet—which had vacuum lines all around the couch!

News Flash: I'm sleeping so much, if I had a corduroy pillow, I'd be making headlines! Ha.

The Good News:

My 17-day period has ended. Will she or won't she? That's the question....

I'm in weekly counseling.

I still have the majority of my eyebrows.

My vision is getting better.

Two weeks ago I was able to watch DVDs (no eye pain or nausea).

Thanks for your love and support.

Love,

Claudia

Natalie: My financial advisor. When she called in the spring to schedule my quarterly appointment with her, I'd just been diagnosed. She immediately offered food help from her church marrieds group (who didn't know anything about me, and were half my age). Weekly, she'd deliver a bag of food from the group. I dubbed this group, "Containers of Love."

Dear Natalie,

May I add to the pancake request something like those applesauce cups—anything but peaches—I'm peached out. The cups count as a "liquid"!! Thanks so much.

Funny—I've been receiving wonderful, deep cards from the group. When I got this from one of the guys, I burst into tears: "I'm on the way to the grocery store and figure I'll cook, and get you well. Deal!"

Have a good day,

C

§

Are you too young to remember "Twiggies"? Twiggy (the model) used to paint on lower eyelashes—looked a bit like a spider crawling across one's face until one learned how to do it artfully. I have some highly embarrassing photos from the late 60s . . . .

Love and good wishes,

Jenny et al. XXXXXXXX

§

Dear Allan,

Thanks for your calls. Maybe this weekend will be better?

Seems your calls fall on my low weeks.

Chapter 15

I often get to the phone while someone is leaving a message if I've not planned ahead to have the phone next to me (also, really, there are a few people I don't even know that well, who are just too fake-happy for my taste right now. Eek. I guess, screening calls?)

C

§

Will give it a go this weekend. Also I understand if you just can't be bothered picking up. Not a problem. At least I know I'm not screened-out for being in the too happy category!!

Allan

§

Dear Marilyn,

Last night's dream: I'm desperately trying to float in a huge lake. My back's arched as far as I can possibly get it—yet I'm almost vertical in the water, my legs dangling below. I'm exhausted, but know I must keep trying to float. Water's lapping over my face. The lake's crowded with plenty of people, but no one seems to notice me. Those geographically closest are oblivious to my struggle.

I awoke able to reflect immediately. Bottom line I took from this dream: My head's still above water and maybe people geographically closest see my strength, not the struggle.

C

§

Your dream said it all. You are keeping afloat! I know that you are having a tough ride. Deep sensitivities are amazing to live with and work with. Let's know together that this experience is deeply healing you on all levels. In consciousness you are already free from the cancer. This freedom is manifesting in your world of experience right now. So it is!

Love,

Marilyn

Chapter 15

Tips for Him or Her:

✔ Ask someone who's sick to visit another time. At this point, your immune system is really compromised.

✔ Keep a surgical mask in your possession, even if it's not "flu season." Use it in stores, especially if crowded. Or if you're in places where debris could blow. I'd almost immediately catch a cold from a breeze—not a gust of wind. The mask looked goofy, but it allowed me to sit in the sun, go to the store, and complete chemo without any delays.

✔ Have the on-call doctor's phone number handy. It'll take too much energy to look for it when you need it. (For me, the need was usually Saturday night.) If you feel you have a fever, take your temperature. If you don't have a thermometer, buy one. If your temperature's above 100.5 go to the emergency room. During weekday hours, call your oncologist.

Tips for Those Who Want to Help:

✔ Follow through. If you say you'll do something, do it. If something comes up and you can't do it, get someone else to follow through for you. I got an e-mail asking what I needed. I requested some bottled water. They said they'd do it in a few days. I thought, *How odd*. We both live right near the same grocery store. One week later, my friend Mary, picked up the water. Two weeks later—the person who originally offered, e-mailed asking if I still needed the water picked up. I simply replied, "No."

✔ Cancel your plans to visit them if you're not feeling well. Even if it's "just a cold."

Chapter 16

OTHER GREAT FRIENDS

AFTER CHEMO #6 (WEEKS ELEVEN AND TWELVE)

Refried beans, corn tortillas. Mac and cheese. Apples, nectarines, peaches, watermelon. I began eating roast beef after thirty years of this little piggy having none. Don't fight what you crave. I just went with the flow of my desires—especially if out of the norm.

Adding variety to my life, I mixed 7-up (flat) with cranberry juice, or had cranberry juice greatly watered down, water, Boost (half a bottle at a time), or carrot juice—in small amounts.

§

I began to consider my couch as a close friend. It was always there—supporting and comforting me hours on end. My "other" friends continued to gently shine for me in various ways. Much of it was behind the scenes—hanging out while I slept, taking out trash, putting up with my mood. How fortunate I am to have these people in my life!

§

One day, looking up at cumulus clouds, the fluffy type that look like sheep, I was immediately transported to some foreign land, absolutely lost in it. My two-minute "trip" was the most wonderful distraction I'd had in months. What a gift to get out, see beauty and be transported!

§

At this point I was complaining a lot, and doing so brought me down. What really seemed to set me off was when someone really cheerful called me. It was like they didn't have a clue (and to be honest, the super cheerful ones didn't). These were the ones who thought being ridiculously "up" and saying catch phrases like, "It's all attitude" and "Be positive" was helping me.

A friend's friend made a bizarre attempt to cheer me up. This extremely perky woman always started with, "You sound so strong! You sound great!" I wanted to clobber her. I hated these cheery calls from this woman, oblivious to my disconnect and low energy level. I listened to myself affirm and argue for my limitations, answering her quiz-like questions one after the other. "I'm tired." "I'm nauseous." I became more morose as she ramped up her perky 'tude. My answers shifted from words to syllables. "Mmm." "Ehh" "Oh." I didn't want to be anyone's project. After her third call I prepared my plea for this woman to concentrate her efforts on world peace, and not on me. She never called again. A friend of mine (who gave this woman my number) suggested to her that the cheerleading go elsewhere.

Then there's the other side. A call telling me about someone I don't know whose implants leaked, causing all sorts of trouble. That same week another person told me, "Be careful about chemo. My friend had troubles after chemo with—"

I interrupted, "That's not supportive. I need support right now."

I still wasn't reading, but was able to watch videos at this point. I only found two comedies funny, so opted for travel videos, and movies from the 1930s and 1940s.

§

Christine called me. "I didn't see you at chemo on Wednesday."

"I was feeling awful, having a meltdown, and slept much of my session." I told her about my emergency room visit. She told me she ended up in the emergency room with a collapsed lung!

Holy Shmoly.

§

A friend in San Francisco called. "I'm coming to San Diego. Let's get together for dinner!" I suggested lunch — and that he bring it to my place. Then I explained why. (He didn't know I had cancer.) We were talking about support, lack of it, spiritual views, and reactions. Right then, two missionaries came to my wide-open door. We waved to each other then I pointed to the phone. I told my friend, "You know, I really am getting support from all corners of the world and spiritual views: USA, New Zealand, Australia, France, Turkey. I've got Agnostic, Christian, Jewish, Muslim, and "Spiritual Leftists" cheering me on. Having these missionaries show up at my door brings my attention to the solace I do get."

§

My friend Rev. John came up from San Diego one day. The people who didn't see me frequently seemed to think I was doing better than I felt at that point.

"What can I do?" John asked.

"Could you please get lunch meat from the deli to make sandwiches, or pull out the frozen dinners from the freezer?"

"What do you want? What would be best for you?" He repeated these when I didn't answer. I was famished and tired. My brain too fried from chemo to think. It's known as "chemo fog." A thick, heavy cloud. Decisions become arduous. Details and questions take too much energy. John is playful and polite. His questioning came from the aspect of care, but I needed him to decide this simple choice rather than toss it back to me repeatedly.

I said, "Shut up" (a phrase I don't use). He did. I could tell he was shocked and hurt. Now I felt nauseous from hunger, more tired from useless conversation, and ashamed of how I was treating my friend. After a few minutes, he asked, "Should I heat up the frozen dinners?"

"Please."

"Do you want the chicken enchilada, or butternut squash?" His not understanding the fog that engulfed me led me to the couch. I sat crying. Finally. Lunchtime. It could've been comical—we were the two least likely people to be found eating frozen, processed meals.

After lunch, I asked him to wash and shred lettuce for me. I never thought I'd have to show someone how to shred lettuce! With a head of iceberg lettuce in one hand, and my plastic, serrated lettuce knife in the other, I gave a demo, making one thin slice. "Just do that a bunch of times." I questioned my idea of having him come up to help save my energy. Once I walked him through shredding, we were fine. It made my "tacos" possible! Melted, pre-shredded cheese on a soft corn tortilla, then I'd add John's

Chapter 16

shredded lettuce, some tomato and a blop of plain yogurt. Without the pre-shredded part, my tacos wouldn't have happened.

Per my list of things to do, John also made Krusteaz pancakes for me to have as snacks or for breakfast the next day. I had him pull a bar stool over to the stove for me. I showed him how to wait until the pancakes were ready for flipping. After this, I was flat-out exhausted. I dove onto the couch, not explaining, or wondering where he'd sit. (I'm a minimalist. The choices aren't comfortable if the couch is taken.) I awoke to find John resting on the floor. He'd waited for me to wake up before leaving—putting him in traffic the entire way home.

§

My friend Rev. Mike (MC) came down from Los Angeles to take me to my doctor's appointment, chemo, counseling and the immune shot the following day. He planned to leave Los Angeles after traffic, with an estimated time of arrival 11 p.m. I told him I might be in a deep sleep if I took the anti-anxiety medication before bed. I heard him arrive, and came out to greet him. Not until after he left the following afternoon did I realize I came out wearing only my blue knit hat, a T-shirt, and underwear—forgetting to further cover my near-bare butt! The next time he called, I apologized for the casual dress code.

He laughed, "I don't recall a hat, but did notice some long, tan legs."

E-mail Updates
To: Bcc
Date: Aug 13

> *Leaving my counseling session, I ran into a man I knew from church in 1991. He moved and got a PhD. In 2000 he came back to church to teach a class, "how to help*

people with cancer." He's now the director at the cancer clinic for psychology programs, co-director of other services, and associate professor of psychiatry. After 10 years of not seeing each other, he recognized me right away—even without my hair! (Somehow that amazes me.) I stood there crying. I told him my energy was really low, so I decided between makeup or getting dressed. "Claudia, You made the right decision."

My counselor tells me I'm well adjusted, and have great coping mechanisms. She's studying mind-sets of people going through cancer, and we both agree I have an edge.

Last week I began a medication meant to prevent chemo side effects—and got a side effect of "jumpy legs" during chemo. This week my oncologist changed the meds.

Neulasta, the after chemo shot, causes excruciating leg pain for four days. I'm told the pain will be less with each shot—two more. (The nurse giving me the shot rolled her eyes when I told her that.) The doctor told me to monitor, but not worry about fever/chills unless they're four days after chemo. Up to that time, fever is a reaction to chemo, not an infection. The doctor's convinced if we switch back to the Neupogen shot, I'd become sick and have to postpone chemo. I've been adamant about nothing getting in my way. I'm going straight through this.

As I write this, I feel the "flu like" feeling creeping up my body/head/throat/eyes. Time to take my temperature, and up to four days after chemo (Saturday) it's OK to take Tylenol. On the fifth day, no more Tylenol, and if I have a temperature, go to the emergency room. Geez! Keep the calendar handy!

Chapter 16

It was a blessing to sleep the first two months through all this. Now I have more energy, so I'm napping about 2-3 hours a day versus napping 8-9 on top of eleven hours sleep. My nails hurt, but are still on; they're in pretty good shape. My hands and feet go numb off/on. My teeth are very sensitive, and my face has gone a bit red/blotchy, but maybe like the gray phase it'll pass quickly. Mouth sores come and go—it's a toss up between drying out the mouth with salt and baking soda to rid mouth sores, or keeping the mouth moist with Biotene toothpaste/mouthwash, ridding dry mouth (which causes cavities).

My friend, Christine, has approached this from a very different angle than me. She's had a glass of wine (and felt sick afterwards), drinks coffee daily (in spite of upset stomach), has people over—cooking for them at times (even if confusing cayenne pepper for paprika). She pushes herself, and is totally open to using prescribed meds to perk her up or calm her down. I baby my stomach (which has virtually no lining), fall asleep at the thought of a nap, and if you've been here, you know how to cook, and where to take the trash—and I thank you!!!! She and I talked about our different styles. We both agree maybe it's because she has an eight-year-old son, and maybe it's her husband who seems to need the support. She has a much more aggressive type of cancer, Her2. She thinks she'll be on a mild type of chemo every month for the rest of her life. So, while I can't even think of deep-sea fishing, she's willing to give it a go (even though later wishing she hadn't)!

I haven't been sick once. No cold, no vomiting, ER visits have sent me home both times within three hours. So, while this has been a DRAG, I've gone through it with WAY more ease than many do, and I give much credit to my support system for that. Thank you. The friends I have all over the world I would not trade for anything. You are golden!

Thanks dear Mark for taking a day off work (and he'll do it again) to cook, clean and quietly hang out with me. He very gently massaged my jumpy leg (a side effect from a drug given to me to prevent side effects from chemo!). No, the massage didn't stop the jumps, but it felt great!

Thanks Mike, for enduring some rocky days of friendship early on, and for twice taking off work to drive three hours from Los Angeles to make me laugh, boost my confidence, do some grocery shopping, and eat meals with me. And most of all, growing through this with me. I went in public with my baldhead for the first time with Mike, but I brought the hat for the on/off chill of shade and air conditioning. When I put on a frilly top and dangly earrings maybe I'll take a photo of what bald confidence looks like. (I think ya gotta do the frilly stuff to feel okay about going bald, though!) This photo has "painted on" eyebrows to fill in the gaps. Leave it to a construction worker gone minister to tell a bald woman, "You look great!"

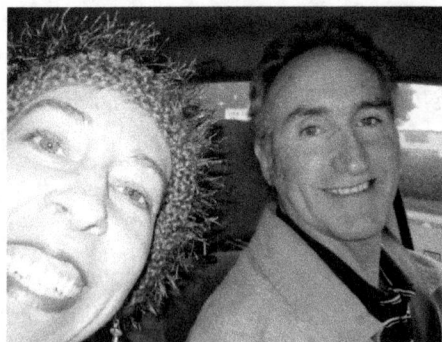

Mike taking me to chemo in August

Chapter 16

§

Dear Claudia,

So relieved to read the latest update. You sound (and look) much more like yourself. The penultimate update had us worried, especially after you had been assured the second round would be easier. What wonderful generous souls your "stable" of good-looking guys are!

Jenny et al.

§

As is usual for me, I have been meaning for at least a month to send a wee package but I seem to have this aversion to Post Offices. Is there anything you want/need—possum gloves/scarf or should that read is there anything you want/need possum-gloves/scarf.

Think about it and let me know.

Cheers,

Allan

§

Sorry you had a rough day. I suspect that you are suffering more from cabin fever and the frustration of not having the energy to do anything about it. Please try not to judge yourself so harshly. As to re-gifting. I see nothing wrong with paying it forward as long as it has no stains, after shave aroma, etc.

Will talk soon. Wish we lived closer so I could annoy you in person.

Keep your chin up!

xx

MC

§

Oh man, my favorite ice cream!! Who is selling our ice cream?

Sweet peas: I cursed your sweet peas for some years cos pink ones kept appearing in random spots, but I actually looove them. I grow 2 big pots of them with bamboo poles in teepee shape for them to grow up. Of course at times the wind blows the whole lot over, pot and all. The weather is great: Warm, early spring. There must be some foul stuff still in store—watch this space.

Movies! . . . I'll keep you posted if more come to mind.

Gotta go do some stuff. Bit tired now.

Cheers,

Allan

§

Dear Allan,

Hokey Pokey ice cream: I guess I'm over it. 3x as sweet as the type I like here. But interestingly, it has more calcium?! 22% vs our 8%. My friend paid $3.00 US for a pint 473 ml. I'm not sure what profit NZ could make for this price. It was only at one store, and they only had a few. Strange, really. What an odd thing to import/ export!

Movies: Oh my—I'm interested in HAPPY movies. The one about the guy murdering his friend sucked. Did you know the same creator made another movie about guys on the run . . . . You might enjoy it! I've heard the one about tough guys living in poverty never moves out of depressing—not up for that. I was thinking light, fun, comedy. Prison breaks? Murder? Violence and poverty?!

Chapter 16

Eek. Well, I'll just stick with travel videos. I've never seen the others you mentioned, but I'm a bit nervous looking further into your list. Ha.

I've been in an on/off pissy mood lately. I'd like to say it is the cancer or steroids, but really I think I'm just fed up with it all and have too much time to think up things to worry about.

Later Al E. Gator,

C

§

Why wouldn't you be pissy? Think about it, and you are actually doing really well. Can you come up with something you want to do when you feel better like go to NY? Can you use my money [sent as gift for half payment of trip to New Zealand] and go to some sort of spa in the desert for a few days? Do you have the energy and eyes to check out that sort of thing on the Internet? How much is it to Norway or Sweden? Why don't you turn your mind to ways you can spend my money?? No I haven't won Lotto but money is only money.

Telling me my taste sucks (movies) — Ha! No one dies in the movie. It's light and has a happy ending.

You wait, Hokey Pokey [ice cream] is gonna be big in the states one day.

Last night after I sent the e-mail telling you about the good weather I checked the TV news. Today's forecast: Gale force northerlies.

Nearly got the package together.

Cheers,

Allan

§

Are you not able to get into the Jacuzzi?

How does sitting near it help?

Karen

§

Dear Karen,

It takes way too much energy to get in/out of Jacuzzi—dress/shower/re-dress . . . . If I'm cold, I either sit in the sun, or dangle my legs in the Jacuzzi. My body's thermostat is very short. I'm cold, then all of a sudden I'm roasting. It's really just an excuse to get outside. There are chairs, sunshine and usually a short conversation with someone walking past. My 5 min walk today ended up being a 7 min walk. I needed to sit on one of those green boxes covering electrical wires that you see along the roads. After a few minutes I continued back to my place. Better than a poke in the eye with a sharp stick, eh?!

Aren't my e-mails uplifting? Ha.

C

§

To: Bcc
Date: Aug 26

Two more chemo days to go. Wow. It sounds really easy putting it that way, but in the next four weeks the drugs will continue to compound.

Until this week I'd been marooned in my apt for 3 wks (except for Dr. appts.) This place is driving me nuts! I'm out for a short time and get fever/chills, then a cold or

Chapter 16

sore throat for two days. My 10 min walks have become occasional 5 min walks. I had this great idea to do errands with a friend. We got in her car, and by the time we got to Costco (3 miles away) I was exhausted. So, like a loyal family dog, I waited in the car as "we" did a few errands. After Mary lugged in the water, juice and fruit, I slept for two-and-a-half hours on the couch.

My pulse is 60; my blood pressure is 80/54. If I'm not having a hot flash, I'm cold, so I sit near the Jacuzzi, just a 30-second walk from my door. The only other person out there is a guy who just returned from Afghanistan (temps 115+).

I was at the clinic getting my blood drawn when an intern who is often in on my exams saw me and said, "Hi." It made me laugh. It was good to know I was recognized with clothes on!

My doctor said my labs were too low this time. He wanted to re-test to see if I could do chemo or not. So, I had a redraw of my blood. (I thought maybe this time they'd use crayons!) We waited an hour to see if I "passed." I did! I got to go ahead with chemo as originally planned. This was a huge blessing. Not missing any treatments means I can get to the other side of all this without delay. It was a very long day as you can see in the photo of Mom and me after eight hours at the clinic. (At least I get to lie in a bed.) Mom stayed with me for the next 36 hours. I'm numb these days, mostly in the chin area—feels like I've been to the dentist. (Tell me if I'm drooling, OK?) Also in the fingers, hands, and feet off/on. The day of chemo feels like my fingers have been slammed shut in a drawer. A day or two later the feeling changes to that tingly sensation you get after running really cold hands under warm water. Ziplock bags are a hassle when fingers are numb! My fingernails are turning dark, but they've stayed on. They look like "smoker's nails" without any smokin'. Then 3-4 days after chemo, I'm still ridiculously bloated and nauseous, then crazy bone (not to be confused with funny-bone) pain takes over for the next 3-4 days, mostly at night.

Sept 9 is my last chemo. Sept 10 my last Neulasta shot. I meet with the surgeon Sept 14. I guess that's when I learn my surgery date.

What fun have YOU had this summer?

Here are some highlights from my "stay-cation"

[Apple's Photo Booth]

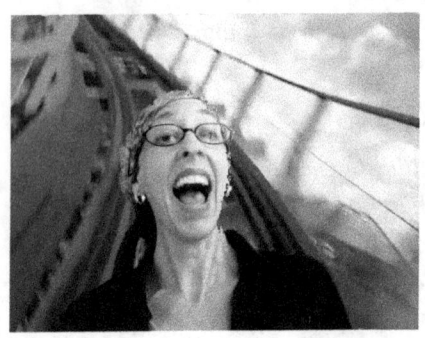
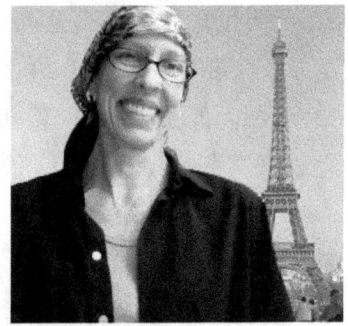
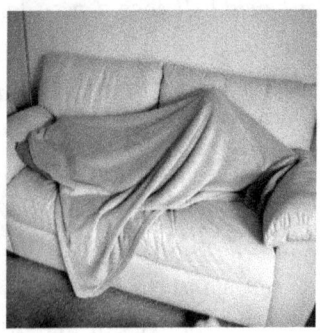

Love, Claudia

PS: "The best way to forget your troubles is to wear tight shoes." ~ Swedish proverb

§

i know you can, i know you will, every day in every way get better and better. . . but it is a RUGGED road, man!!! i'm sad it is so very rugged . . . but you, my dearest, are a beautiful trooper.

big hug to all those helping you, biggest hug to nancy.

LOVE LOVE LOVE

Michele

Tips for Those Who Want to Help:

✔ Offer to go to a cancer clinic class, meeting or any social event with them.

✔ Instead of continuously asking, "Where's this go." "Where would I find . . . ?" Open up drawers and cupboards. Look around. You're there to help. You're not snooping.

✔ Take their car to a car wash.

✔ Ask if they want to go somewhere with you, or be left alone to nap while you're gone.

✔ Read to them if their vision is affected by chemo, or if they're too tired to read. I loved when people read me a page or two from an uplifting book or a daily devotional reading.

✔ Encourage them to drink liquids. Offer a drink or something moist to eat. If their throat hurts or feels swollen, they need to swallow more. Pudding, Jell-O, popsicles, milkshakes, soup, broth, fruit cups, applesauce—they all count as liquids. At this stage, it's more appealing to see two tablespoons of pudding instead of a bowl of it. This isn't the time to bring home a Big Gulp to show you care about their hydration. Besides, soda and hot drinks don't aide in hydration as well as other choices. Offer to split a fruit cup, or pour them a small drink–pour yourself one, too. We're social beings. We eat and drink more around others. Remind them to take sips throughout the day instead of drinking all at once, or right before a meal (which will fill them up, taking away any desire to eat).

Chapter 17

EMERGING FROM THE FOG

AFTER CHEMO #7 (WEEKS THIRTEEN AND FOURTEEN)

I made my first meal. Mac and cheese. (You know, boil the water, add the mystery packet of cheese, milk and butter.) I sat on a barstool during the process and was exhausted. But I made my first meal.

Spinach lasagna. Cold baked beans on toast (something I hadn't thought of since living in New Zealand eleven years ago). Apples, nectarines, pears, bananas, watermelon. Activia yogurt. Frozen pancakes or waffles. Roast beef sandwich, hot dogs (cold from the refrigerator, or cooled down after being microwaved). Corn on the cob—I let it cool down to room temperature. After thirteen weeks of no interest in sweets, I was enjoying a bite of cake here, a cookie there, and flan. The same drinks as usual, plus Ovaltine with room temperature water.

§

Psst! Every orifice in my body made noise after Wednesday (chemo day) through the next week or so. I was so bloated I could care less what it sounded like, or from where it came! It usually went something like this (No, I'm not going to describe the sounds for you!): Wednesday and Thursday: Bloated, nauseous, and on a liquid diet. Tired, yet amped up from steroids. Friday, Saturday: Bloated and constipated (more so on Taxol chemo than on Adriamycin and Cytoxan). Fever, flu-like aches. My eyes were dry, fatigued and watered easily. My stomach hurt, so I took antacid pills. I had two days of near-constant restless leg syndrome. I wasn't up for company.

The Saturday night after Taxol, bone pain set in. Sleep was almost impossible. Neulasta, the shot I received in my stomach the day after chemo, helped the body make more white blood cells—which helped the body prevent infection. The frequent and random pain was excruciating in my feet, ankles, legs and occasionally my pelvis, arms, and back. On Taxol, nausea was less intense, but constant. Before, on Adriamycin and Cytoxan, I had severe nausea from Wednesday (chemo day) to Monday, and a few times in the following week.

E-mail Updates

> *Those beautiful blue eyes are still as blue as the mighty Pacific on a clear day. Karen*

§

> *Thanks for the update. Just one more chemo to go. I know you will be glad when it's over. I hope the bump in your left breast turns out to be nothing. I loved your stay-cation photos. They were great!*
>
> *I love you!*
>
> *Dad*

§

Rev. John: We met at a church meeting in 2000 and have been friends since. He's now the senior minister of San Diego Center for Spiritual Living, CA.

Chapter 17

Blessings of Love,

Wholeness and Light my dear friend!

Namaste,

John & Connie

§

So how was Paris?

Don't feel bad about Ziploc bags — I'm often challenged when it comes to sealing those wretched things. Second only to no-name Saran wrap . . . .

You are brave to even think about going to Costco. It's a major adventure for us, and one only undertaken very occasionally. Prescriptions mostly. Rarely find the need for a pallet of Cheetos, which is the type of thing so many customers at our local one seem to be buying. That and enormous Christmas/Halloween decorations; really curious where they store things like that off season . . . .

Good luck this week (and always). We are thinking of you.

Love,

Jenny

Tips for Those Who Want to Help:

✔ Call or e-mail asking if they need anything. Give them a reasonable time when you'll come by so they don't spend their energy waiting.

✔ Get the mail. Take out the garbage. Bring in the empty garbage cans. Rake leaves. Suggest a child draw a picture, make a card, or help with age-appropriate chores.

✔ Check in briefly—but more than a drop and dash. Depending on my day, ten to twenty minutes was a good time to visit with someone who wasn't part of my core support team.

✔ Invite them to a party, a visit or lunch. Don't confuse their being tired with not wanting to be included. On your turf, offer a bed or couch for a nap. Or offer them to stay the night. Let them decide if they can join you—even if for a quick appearance.

✔ Look around and ask if there's anything you can do before leaving.

✔ If they have flowers, check if the flowers need fresh water, or trashing.

✔ Be aware of their energy level. Park close to store entrance. Pump gas for them. Offer to push the grocery cart—or let them push it if the cart gives them support.

✔ Carry things. Load and unload the car. Put things away and let them know where you've put them.

Chapter 18

CHIN OVER THE BAR

AFTER CHEMO #8 (WEEKS FIFTEEN AND SIXTEEN): LAST ONE!

White beans, black beans and pinto beans. While not a complete protein, I craved them. I was tired of other carbohydrates—and they were everywhere. Potatoes, bread, and now small amounts of cookies and cake were back on the scene. The taste for drinks remained the same as the previous few weeks.

§

Every two weeks, my oncologist asked, "Are you doing self-exams?"

"No."

On the third appointment (six weeks into chemo) I said, "I can't stand the idea of you hitting your head against the wall, so I'm answering, 'Yes.'"

In September, two weeks before my chemo treatments ended, I answered with, "I found a lump last week during self-examination on the other side."

The following week I had an ultrasound of the new finding. The doctor (who was new to me) asked three times when I was starting chemo. I had a scarf on my head. No wig. No hair of any sort to be seen. I finally, slowly said: "I-do-not-have-hair. My-last-chemo-is-next-week." He scheduled me with someone else for my biopsy. I'm sure it had nothing to do with the tone of our conversation.

After being really worked up over this guy—who said, "I've been doing this for sixteen years." I decided to shift my attitude from: What did this doctor think? I had a scarf on my head, and just happened to be in the cancer clinic? To: The guy thought I looked great!

His comment about "doing this for sixteen years" came after I started to cry. With the ultrasound wand he kept going back to the site of the bump, then showed me the image of the dark, strange shape on the monitor.

"It's not cancer. Trust me."

I didn't.

§

On Labor Day I was wearing long pants, a long sleeve shirt, wool sweater, silk scarf around my neck, and a knit hat. It was 78 degrees and I was cold. (Until the hot flashes ignited, then I couldn't get the layers off quick enough!) I was trying to convince myself that my white blood cell count would be high enough for my last chemo that Wednesday. I'd gone back to sleeping twelve hours and napping two to four more. There was something to be said about sleeping my way to health! Being awake and not able to do anything was downright crazy. My hands were numb with neuropathy.

§

Second week in September: LAST CHEMO! I just about crawled to my oncology appointment. I got the news, "Your white

Chapter 18

cell count is too low for chemo. Let's take another blood draw to see if your numbers have gone up since yesterday." After having a tube of blood taken, I waited for results. Curling up in a chair is something little girls look cute doing. At age forty-four and five feet eight inches with a fused spine, it looks pathetic. I was told, "If your numbers are close to 1,500 you can do chemo as planned." I got to move forward with 946. I guess "close" is relative. In general terms, 1,500 is considered mild neutropenia, and a mild risk for infection.

Done! The nurse unplugged the I.V. from my port. I just sat there. No bells, whistles, or flashing lights. For a moment, I felt the weight lifted. Chemo's over. I wept in relief for the journey coming to an end. I wept for the journey not even half over. (I'd have a biopsy the next day for my left breast, and a mastectomy pre-op appointment the following week for my right.)

Every time I hear of someone who's walked this path before me, especially if they died of cancer, I bless them. My path was easier because they forged before me. *Thank you, and God's blessings to you.*

§

Mike and Allan, two of my dear friends who don't know each other—but both know I back down to very little, each shared with me they were silently concerned I'd walk away from chemo before, or during. Both of these friends later said, "—But you did it." And, "You completed chemo."

Funny. Chemo was finished—and yet not really. Thursday, Friday and Saturday I was still extremely bloated, nauseous, and numb, and had leg pain, spasms, and surging hot flashes. So, when does one celebrate? Is it at the last chemo? Is it when the next chemo would have been—and isn't? After surgery? And if so, which surgery? Tumor removal? Reconstruction? And which one— Implants? Nipples? When the energy's back? (I'm told it takes one to two years to regain energy, though some say it takes longer.)

What I knew then was, I sure don't have any. I must admit, four days after the fact, I was closer to feeling the thrill of it being done than I was on the Wednesday of my last chemo. I saw the light at the end of the tunnel. I was pretty sure it wasn't a train.

Tips for Him or Her:

✔ Wear patterned tops, and tops with texture to camouflage the expansion and reconstruction process. Rectangular scarves hanging down like a tie, or draped off to one side gave me confidence that the whole world wasn't focused on "One-eyed Betty." Using iron-on sparkles or patches (there are tons of designs!) also camouflages an erect nipple.

✔ When you complete treatment—whether it is radiation, chemo, or whatever, take a moment to honor what you've done. You don't need to wear it on your sleeve, but do acknowledge yourself, and all who've helped you. Give thanks to God, others, and yourself. You have made it through one hell of a journey.

✔ Look at the types of food you've gotten in the habit of eating for quick meals and calories. Now it's time to think about what you'll cook for yourself, and what it'll look like on your body.

Tips for Those Who Want to Help:

✔ Let someone go in front of you at the store (even without cancer).

✔ Send or bring a care package—it doesn't have to be expensive: A satin pillowcase, scarves, gum, an eyebrow pencil, Biotene mouthwash or toothpaste, lip balm, music, book (they may or may not be able to read it right away), T-shirt, necklace, simple food (think child-friendly textures, tastes), postage stamps, etc.

Chapter 19

E-MAIL CELEBRATIONS

To: Bcc
Date: Sept 10
LAST CHEMO DONE!!!!!!!!!

> *My sore, numb feet, hands and face will begin to heal. The bone pain has had its last three-day run, and my white-coated tongue will soon enjoy the taste of food again! I'm told in about three weeks I'll see my thick eyebrows begin to grow back, and hair will begin sprouting up again on my head!!*

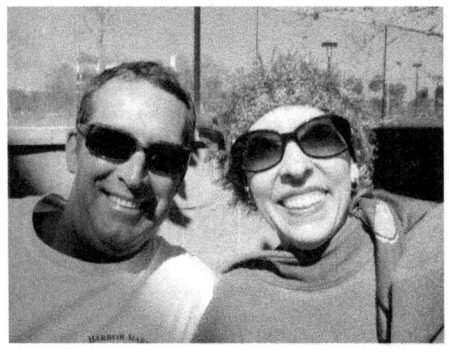

Thanks for prayers, cards, e-mails, transportation, shopping/preparing and cutting watermelon, etc. For putting up with a range of moods, being willing to stand on your head if that would make me happy, coming over to sleep on my couch while I slept in bed. It's all the DOING you have done that has allowed me to sleep, and trust all is taken care of. With heartfelt appreciation, thanks a million.

Keep in touch, keep the faith, and keep on keeping on.

Love,

Claudia

§

YEAH!

I Celebrate Your Blessings

of Spiritual Trust and Tenacity!

Namaste,

Rev John

§

Dear Allan,

"Pineapple lumps"—gee, I'm glad I'm not hyper sensitive to "LUMPS." I mean, I seem to have plenty right now. I thought, eek. Pineapple? But you're right—things don't taste the same, so I gave it a go—and I've eaten half the package!

I LOVE that bear! He really looks like a rugby player! He's got the Haka moves down, ready to teach Kamaputu! [Another bear Allan gave me when I lived in New Zealand.]

Chapter 19

I know the package cost you a fortune. Sorry. Believe me, it's well worth it! But now I better understand your aversion to the post office.

My hands are too numb to enjoy the scratchers [lotto] today, but I figure in a few days I'll be rich-rich-rich!!! (I'll let you know!) Anything over $10,000 we'll go 50/50. Really, I'd have been thrilled to just get scratchers in a card—but I must say you put together great care packages.

Well, interesting, after my Dr appt, my friend Christine called to congratulate me on completing chemo last week. I told her my Dr appt results from today. She was happy for me. She wishes they'd do a bi-lateral mastectomy on her. She said, "Hey man, this way, it'll never get you again." Wow. A bit drastic, but true. She also said, "Now you'll be even!" She asked for a bilateral, and they wouldn't give her one, as she has one healthy side (even though her cancer is more aggressive than mine). So, it was really nice to have her (perverse) view of celebration for me. I have appt with plastic surgeon this Thurs, and will know more then.

Thanks again.

Love,

C

§

Thanks for the phone call. I saved it and played it a couple of times. Na it's not the money-believe me it doesn't even occur to me. I thought it was you who taught me that the universe will provide?? Strange as it may seem to you, I actually work full time and hence the $ becomes relative to what you are earning. I know some of the things may not be appropriate-maybe lip balm or some such thing-who knows what might irritate or not. Glad you like the bear-I was quite taken with him. Just remember the Haka is like a challenge. Whatever the literal words mean, and they are a bit strange, it says to the world: Bring it on, I'll handle it and come out on top. And you will. I know the news is a bit tough but you will get through.

Oh, and I can't believe your memory for Carlos. Carlos Spencer was an All Black [New Zealand Rugby] and I think he did underwear ads eg him just in knickers or boxers, looking quite spunky (or so the girls told me).

Catch ya soon,

Allan

§

Dear Allan,

Spencer!!! I remember the cookie commercial where a wife and her husband are sitting on the couch, watching TV and eating cookies. With each bite she "sees" her husband who is on the couch in his bathrobe—fat and comfy—as Carlos in his bathrobe—toned and scrumptious. It was funny.

Ah-Ha. Things in box that may not be appropriate. Yes. Thank goodness I decided to read. I thought the manuka honey (bath stuff) was something to eat! Lip balm I thought how smart of you—I have used lip balm every day for 4 months. Sniff box—lavender seems to be the only smell I've been able to handle, so thanks for not sending me other smells. See? You really do a great job at care packages! Cute tea towels. That must mean paper plates and plastic utensils are near an end!

Chapter 19

Haka. Nice insight re: challenge, bring it on I can handle it. I think you should get Skype or FaceTime working so you can see the bear do the Haka. He's quite good at it!

Anyway, thanks for the vote of confidence. I don't know if I'm numb, or just (almost) ready for surgery. I didn't have the absolute meltdown like I had the first time. Funny, maybe people aren't fully reading my updates. I got two e-mails saying how happy they were for me. I venture to say it was re: chemo ending, and they skimmed over the surgery part, or thought it was a double anyway, who knows?

Guess what I'm going to try to do today? A yoga class for bald women! Or should I say, those of us with promise of re-growth. I hope we do an hour of Shavasana—that pose where you just lie there real still.

I saw a photo of me right before chemo with thick eyebrows. I realized how much mine have thinned out. Paint-on-eyebrows just don't cut it for me. I hope they grow back thick again.

Well, that's it from here.

C

§

Yay! No more chemo!!! Phase 1 is behind you—that is a victory. It may not feel like one everyday, but it is a huge victory.

My friend Carrie dropped off some food for you this afternoon—crackers, fruit salad and some pasta. Is there anything else I can get for you this week?

Best,

Natalie

§

Dear Natalie,

When I left Thurs I was so wiped out. Thanks for listening, and thanks for the oodles of food I came home with!

When I got home, I immediately ate (most of) the watermelon, some fruit salad, and some cold pasta—all right out of the containers! I do hope my manners return soon. They've gone out the window in the name of saving energy. After inhaling food, I waddled over to the couch and took a nap.

You are a very special lady. Your Light shines so clear and freely.

Love,

Claudia

§

I know it's risky telling you what to do/not do but you can always skip this next sentence cos it gets better after this. Don't let any numbness/pain problems go on without complaining. The docs etc are there to take care of those things.

Start reading again from here.

Thanks for the cards, which arrived yesterday. I'm especially EXCITED by 'Watching the cricket'. I'm going to put it in a frame and it will go on the wall. You no doubt bought it because of the cricket theme but what you don't know is that I LOVE naive art (I don't know if you read the back of the card or if you have heard of naive art but very few have). You see so little of it. I

Chapter 19

think if I had to collect one type of art then that would be it.

Thanks again.

Catch ya soon,

Allan

§

Dear Allan,

Shit. The wrath of Claudia. I'm hearing, things like: I know it's risky telling you what you do/don't want to hear from several angles. Oh well, at least from those who listen! I laughed to read the bold—start reading here.

C

§

Well, you have mellowed a tad since this process began but it still pays to be careful.

The news is good, I'm very happy. Hell, replacement in 12-15 years, not a problem. I think I'll have hips and knees replaced by then. Don't be tolerant of the pain. That's what meds are for: To cover it up while you've got it. It'll go but why suffer in the meantime. And hey sleeping ain't a problem. It's good if you are awake to pee/poo and eat. That's it, anything else is a bonus . . . .

Allan

§

As always, easy for me to say, but I'm hopeful that the pain and discomfort will be better than from the chemo. My attitude is that it's up to the medicos to make sure I don't have pain. That's what drugs are for. Make sure *you tell 'em when you are hurting and that they do something about it. I honestly don't think there is any need to suffer pain—I know I haven't been down this track personally but I have been involved and my recollection is that this is what the docs themselves said—you tell us what's happening and we'll get the dosage and the mix right.*

If you want me to come over [from New Zealand] just let me know. Might be tough to do for Oct 6 but who knows. If not, then I'm sorry the burden is gonna be on you and your mum. Sometimes you need someone to act as the go-between or advocate with the medical people and looks like that's your mum. If I can't do anything else, use the money for anything to help you through, just please just use it. e.g. more expensive drugs, or tell your mum to order in food to keep you both going, or taxis to pick up a taco, or a flamenco dancer to cheer you both up—whatever. You don't need to check with me. [Allan sent me money for a trip to New Zealand right before my diagnosis.]

Take care,

Allan

Chapter 20

NOW WHAT?

I had an appointment with my surgical oncologist. The meeting began with, "The good news is the biopsy is showing benign. The—"

I interrupted, "—other news?"

"Yes. The other news is . . . ."

Here I am again, six months later, hearing Charlie Brown's teacher: "Whaa-whaa-whaa-whaa-whaa." The ultrasound showed one lump was clearly a cyst. No problem to drain with a needle. The other lump didn't look like a cyst, yet was coming back benign. The doctors were puzzled. They preformed a vacuum type biopsy, taking fifteen sample cores from my left breast. I hurt for over two weeks. The doctor who did the biopsy said he'd call me on Friday with the results. I didn't get a call. I figured he'd had a busy day and forgot. Sure enough.

The surgeon ordered another mammogram to be done "immediately" for my left side. I opted to save time and walk down the hall in my hospital exam gown. My surgeon laughed, but I sensed she was pleased with my time management skills. After the mammogram, I was told, "Wait here until we know the results." I sat in the communal waiting room (the nook where women sit in their gowns, chatting, and turning magazine pages, waiting for their mammogram, ultra sound, biopsy, or results). After twenty-five minutes, I got up and poked my head out into the hallway—

and saw the doctor who did the biopsy last week walking toward me. I knew this wasn't good.

He immediately apologized for not calling me Friday, explaining, "I wanted to talk with your surgeon first. We don't understand how I pumped the vacuum fifteen times to get core samples—and only six samples came out. I didn't want to leave that sort of message with you on a Friday—then I forgot to take your phone number in case I changed my mind—which I did, to call you over the weekend."

At this point I told him my endurance wasn't good for standing, and asked if we could we sit down somewhere and talk. He brought me to the room where they review films. He showed me my mammograms—the ones before and after the ultrasound; both left and right. He phoned my surgeon, asking her to come down the hall to view the mammogram results.

Ugh. Were they going to say I needed another biopsy? No. They were now suggesting a bilateral mastectomy.

They gave me two more options. "You could let it go three months, then come back for another ultrasound, biopsy, mammogram, and possibly surgery to dig out whatever it is. The surgery will disfigure you. The third option is to come back in three months for a mastectomy on the left side." The two doctors were in strong agreement that things weren't okay left alone.

After looking at my options and guessing my best outcome, I opted to move forward just a few weeks away. "I'm not going through any of this again. If you truly have concern, let's do it now." By "it" I meant a bilateral mastectomy. Saying it is one thing. Realizing it's happening is another. My head began to spin.

My surgeon and I walked back to the exam room together. Now I completely understand those who have trouble walking and chewing gum at the same time. In my strategically wrapped gown, carrying my top, sweater and purse, I searched for Kleenex in the back pocket of my jeans, still on me. All while realizing I came in to

Chapter 20

talk about a mastectomy on the right side, and was leaving with paperwork for a mastectomy on both sides.

I've heard stories of woman choosing to have a bilateral even without cancer on both sides. To me, that was nuts! While I wiped mourning tears away, I better understood women opting for a bilateral to ensure never having breast cancer again—and to have matching sides. Just like the first side being diagnosed, the left side was completely off my radar for why I was at the doctor. I felt the shock but didn't have a meltdown. I could absorb the original surgery prep information for which I had the appointment.

When we got back to the exam room I asked the surgeon, "Now what?"

She said, "The surgery prep and procedure is the same—but now on both sides."

I had a hard time wrapping my head around how easy it sounded.

§

Next, I had an appointment with my reconstruction surgeon to ask questions, and to see what an implant looked and felt like. A surgery date was set. During the same surgery the surgical oncologist would remove cancer, both breasts, and as few lymph nodes as possible, if needed. The reconstruction surgeon would put into place the expanders to stretch the skin over the next several months, creating room for the implants. Yes, it feels like it sounds. Ouch. But more on that later.

Tips for Him or Her:

✔ Bring someone with you to appointments if you feel you'll need support hearing unexpected news. You may choose for them to wait for you in the waiting room, or to join you in the exam room. If they join you, you might ask them to take notes.

✔ Tell your doctor you're not ready to make the decision yet if you need time to think a situation through. Be realistic with a time frame.

✔ Bring your own reading material, notes to write, or something else to do in case of office delays, or impromptu medical procedures that involve a waiting room.

✔ Stay as positive and flexible as possible. It really does help.

✔ If you need time alone to process any news, tell family and friends. Some may call wanting an update about your doctor visit.

✔ If you have scans where you receive contrast through your veins, or if you have blood tests, or surgery, sometimes the medical folks want your arm—not your port. If they've had a difficult time getting to your vein in the past, or if it's been extremely uncomfortable, ask them to wrap your arm in a heated blanket for a few minutes before they come at you with the needle. It makes a huge difference for vein accessibility and comfort! Also, drink plenty of fluids one to two days before these procedures to plump up your veins.

Tips for Those Who Want to Help:

✔ When their treatment is over, go easy on interrogation. Questions like, "Did they get it all?" "Are you cancer-free?" can be difficult to answer. Don't ask if you can't handle the answer. If they don't volunteer the information, maybe it's because they're still processing it themselves, or they don't want to affirm cancer. Maybe they're only sharing the information with those they know

Chapter 20

will truly hold them in the Light, and not just quip, "I'll say a prayer for you." I was surprised at how many people who didn't really know me asked my status. I'd give a thumbs up, or say, "Things are great." Sometimes they'd repeat the question, as if insisting to hear, "Yes. I'm cancer free." On occasion, I'd say, "No. I've chosen to live with it at a lower stage, in remission." Casual conversations trailed off with this answer, and I'd usually follow with, "I'm fine, but unless you really know someone, be careful with that question."

Chapter 21

WHERE'S GALLAGHER?

A neighbor was over visiting. My front door was open. A young woman from two doors down, with whom I'd spoken only once, walked by. Then she came back to my open door and whispered, "Claudia" as she curled her index finger toward her. I walked to the door and she pointed to her head, still whispering, "Do you have cancer?"

I laughed and said, "It's okay. No need to whisper. Yes."

She absolutely flipped out. "Oh my God!!"

I wasn't in the mood for comforting someone I didn't know by telling them all my intimate details.

Without invitation, she followed me into my apartment. Continuing to express her shock, "Oh my God! I didn't know!"

"I'm fine." I sat back down, and introduced the two neighbors to each other.

One didn't know how to cut watermelon and preferred to use a paring knife for the job, insisting, "Your knives are too big, and too sharp." (I've had four people freak out over the size and sharpness of my knives!)

The other neighbor kept interrupting my watermelon cutting lesson with questions. "Are you in chemotherapy?"

"I just finished." It was nicer than, No I shaved my head to look like the tenant upstairs. "Do you need a massage? You should come to my spa and get a deep tissue massage."

I asked if she'd ever known anyone with cancer. She said, "Yes."

I'm not sure how well she knew their story. The skin for someone in chemo is so delicate. Avoiding deep tissue massage is the rule I heard. I wasn't up for being quizzed, especially by someone I didn't feel had the right to invade my privacy. This neighbor then started to whine and put on a pouty face to express how sad she was for what I was going through. I don't do well with whiners. "Your whining doesn't help me. Stop it."

My other neighbor, gesturing with the paring knife jumped in, "Look at her! She's always got a smile on her face! She's my hero!"

Then the whiner actually threw herself on me to give me a hug. When people hugged me, their shoulder would often hit my port, causing pain. Angry, I used all my strength to push her away, "Don't hug me. Back off!" I'm a straight-shooter—often to a fault. None of my tone, body language, or words did any good. She hugged me then stepped back.

I said, "You've been really intrusive."

"Oh, I know, the energy thing."

For once I wasn't talking about energy, vibes, or the spiritual realm—and nobody seemed to be getting me! At that point, I felt like leaving them both in my place and if I ended up with pieces of watermelon by way of Gallagher's Sledge-O-Matic method, so be it! "The Hugger" never said hello again, and moved within six months.

§

After counseling I swung by the resource room at the cancer clinic to see what information they had about mastectomies. Several employees and volunteers were standing around. I said, "Whoa. Are you open?"

They laughed and simultaneously said, "Yes!"

Chapter 21

They were making an educational video, and they were thrilled a real patient walked in asking for help. They asked if I'd be willing to be in the video. Of all days! The scarf I wore was my least favorite. It was too small, and silk—needed adjusting throughout the day because silk doesn't stay put like cotton. I agreed to the filming, although self-conscious of my scarf. I told them what I came in for. We discussed the information of a mastectomy while being video taped, without audio.

I left the resource room and headed out to find a mastectomy camisole—a camisole with special pockets for the drains after surgery. It's used for two weeks. I never wore it and ended up having my mom return it. Instead, I wore the "after-surgery bra" put on me immediately after surgery. I found it comfortable. It was snug, and I felt protected. Unless you have a mastectomy camisole with the built-in pockets for drains, the best way around these heavy drains hanging from your body (bad idea) is to safety-pin the drains to the inside of your shirt. I wore a dark blouse or loose fitting shirt and safety-pinned the drains to the inside of the tops. It worked well for me. If you only have one drain, it can hideout in a little sling purse.

On the way home I was tired, and my feet were numb and sore from neuropathy. Just ahead of major traffic, I only needed to step on the brakes a few times. The act of stepping on the break was more analytical rather than feeling the peddle under foot. I arrived home exhausted, and hit the couch immediately.

Oh my gosh! The next day I was so sore. The day before had been a bigger day than I gave myself credit for. I slept twelve hours and my feet still hurt when I woke up. I have so much to do before surgery, two weeks away. I'd like these feet to cooperate! I stayed near the couch, "walking" on my knees if I needed anything. Hobbling for laundry. Sitting to make a meal I've come to call "miracle of cans." Here's my secret recipe: Can of black beans, can of corn, chop some red onion, chop some tomato (or open a can if you have one!). Shake on some cumin, oregano—and on an energetic day, add avocado, maybe chop some celery, and sprinkle shredded cheese on top. Presto! It's dinner! After those two chores I was wiped-out, even eager to collapse into an unmade bed.

§

Once a month, a local team of maids came to my house. "Cleaning for a Reason" is a national program with local agencies that gift monthly house cleaning to women undergoing treatment for breast cancer. I was the first ever recipient for the company serving me. The owner asked if I'd agree to talk with news reporters in exchange for an extra cleaning. I agreed.

The four maids were busy at work when the TV crew arrived. I sat up from the couch to greet the TV crew, then lay back down until they were ready. "How has the cleaning service helped you?"

"Cleaning the floor, tub, toilet and vacuuming are things I don't have strength for now. It means a lot to me. In a way, it's how I can gift those coming to help me—to give them a break from doing one more thing." I motioned to Maids.com on my *wall of gratitude*. The TV crew filmed the list hanging on the wall. "The list guides me to refocus on the good going on in my life."

In the middle of filming, the phone rang. I heard the message being left. I apologized to the crew, saying, "I need to take this." They quit filming and waited for me. The nurse practitioner had an opening the next day. She wanted me to come in, pick up a prescription for neuropathy pain, and see me walk. She said the pain and numbness should go away in about four months, but could be up to a year, maybe two, with most of the progress seen in four months.

The TV crew wanted an action shot. "What will you do after we leave?" I pointed to the couch. One of them saw a watermelon on the counter. Yes, another one. I'm craving watermelons. An added bonus: They count as liquid intake and are high in iron. "Could we get an action shot of you cutting the watermelon?"

Chapter 21

Without hesitation I said, "No." My foremost thought: I'd make the first cut—then what? I'd be left, exhausted, with a mess and holding a knife I couldn't feel in my hand. I was glad when the interview finished. It zapped my energy, in addition to last night's clean up. I'd put away books and piles of papers I have around, especially now in preparation for surgery.

A few days after the TV interview, I called the owner expressing my thanks for his care and help. I asked him to give his payment for an extra cleaning as a bonus to his employees, or the cleaning as a gift to someone else who needed it.

Tips for Him or Her:

✔ Get two safety pins to secure the drains to your clothing if you decide to forego the mastectomy camisole. The drains have a little loop in which you can thread a safety pin.

✔ Limit your time with people who don't "get it." If someone is rough, tell them not to touch you.

✔ Ask people to shred lettuce, cut watermelon, dice chicken, or open things for you. If you can't feel your grip on a knife, explain neuropathy to people when asking for help.

Tips for Those Who Want to Help:

✔ Chop up small amounts of onion, celery or other food for them to have ready in the refrigerator. If they have neuropathy, their fingers, and possibly feet are hot, tingly and numb. If you need to experience it, go slam your fingers in a door to get an idea. If neuropathy is in their feet, offer to do errands, or chores around the house.

✔ Do your whining somewhere else. Some people are taken aback that I don't tolerate whiners. I've been a therapist, counselor, social worker and minster. I can have compassion and empathy, but zero tolerance for drama with no action. To me, whining is worse than worry. Worry can at least be turned around to a positive thought or comment.

✔ No bear hugs or crunching handshakes! During cancer treatment, senses are heightened. A neighbor who had recently entered my life came over to cut watermelon for me. My hands were pretty numb at that point; knives were better given to someone who could feel their grip.

Chapter 22

MY MASTECTOMY - TAKE TWO

Heading to my pre-op appointment, I walked past the radiology department. Cheers spilled into the hallway after a patient rang the brass bell—a sound of victory following someone's last radiation treatment. The cheers gave me goose bumps and brought tears to my eyes. Good for you! I wondered why chemo didn't have some fanfare upon completion. Then I thought, it would take too much effort, be too noisy—and some finish lines look very different. At the end of chemo, I just wanted to go home. I thought it was absolutely grand to have that brass bell at radiation, ringing into the common hallway for all to hear!

At my appointment the surgical oncologist said she couldn't feel any tumors.

"You can't?"

"Can you?"

"Yes." I led her hand.

"Claudia, that's your rib." We both laughed.

I asked, "How many women can do that?!"

The tumors had completely shrunk!

§

The weekend before my surgery I heard a segment on National Public Radio about the New York Burlesque Festival. The teacher, Jo "Boobs" Weldon, said she once had a private class for a woman who'd had a bilateral mastectomy. She taught her to twirl tassels! I paid attention like no other radio show I'd heard. Wow! This woman could do that after a mastectomy?! Things might be okay for me after all. (No, I haven't taken up tassel twirling, but knowing it can be done is a huge shift for me in hope of retuning to normalcy.)

§

I received a call at 3 p.m. the day before surgery. "Your surgery has been moved up from 3 p.m. to 7 a.m.. To save time in the morning, you need to get to the hospital now for a procedure."

"I live twenty-two miles away and traffic has begun."

In a more direct tone, she said, "That's why you need to leave now. Radiology knows you'll be here around 4 p.m.". I dropped everything not really knowing what I was in for. A doctor in radiology injected four radioactive markers into my breast and underarm so the tumors would be easily found both in X-rays and during surgery. Through this radiologist I learned my surgical oncologist was one of the top breast cancer surgeons in Southern California.

§

October 6. I had a bilateral mastectomy. What other way to celebrate OktoberBreast? Beer anyone? It's national breast cancer awareness month, after all. Mary drove me to the hospital. Mom met us there. Surgery went fantastically well! Natalie, my financial

Chapter 22

advisor, arrived with incredible posters as if on cue after my transfer from recovery room to hospital room. She whirled in, jumped up to tape the posters on the wall, then headed back to work. What an awesome thing to focus upon!

One of the posters
Natalie made for me

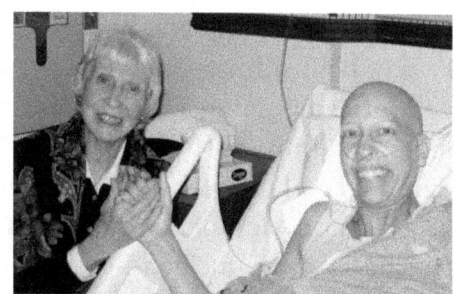

Arm wrestling with my mom?

My mom's calm, strong, and intelligent. People go to her in a crisis. The morning after surgery she telephoned my hospital room. "I'll be there as soon as I get my car out of the shop." When she left the hospital the night before, her nerves were raw. She was wrenched. So was her car. She'd hit a road medium, completely damaging two tires and throwing her car alignment off.

Fortunately, she was okay.

§

Post-op, my every output after I used the toilet was measured. When I saw (I kid you not) glow-in-the-dark poop I said, "Uh . . . what's going on?"

The nurse's jaw dropped. She left, bringing someone back with her. After a long silence, the second nurse figured it out. "Did you go to radiology before surgery?"

"Yes. Ohhhhh. They injected me with radioactive markers." Long ago I worked in a physical rehabilitation center, and I know there were giggles and jokes in the charting room about the bald lady with glow-in-the-dark bowel movement!

I stayed in the hospital until Friday, October 9. At home, my mom and friends took shifts 24/7 for the first week-and-a-half. I needed someone to provide an arm—not so much for strength, but something to hang on to as I got my legs out of bed. (The combo of having both sides operated upon, and having a fused spine left me with little mobility.) These friends also prepared meals, and helped me change my post-surgery dressings. Fed up with the drains, I didn't take photos. The drains come out of the side of the body, rib height. Each side of the body has a tube the diameter of a thick pencil, leading to hand-grenade-looking vessels capturing the draining blood and other body fluid output, which I'd measure twice a day.

For the post-op appointments, I grabbed a big scarf, and a suit jacket that had inside pockets. I felt prettier in this outfit than in any shirt I could get in and out of by myself. (After surgery, raising my arms over my head was rough, and with neuropathy my fingers were too numb for tiny buttons.) I tucked both the scarf and drains into the interior suit pockets, putting each drain in a sandwich bag, just in case they leaked. The surgical oncologist pulled out the hospital gown at the post-op appointment, I said, "Wait. Don't leave. I don't need that." And I unbuttoned the two large buttons on my suit. There I was in the "after-surgery bra" which looks much like a zip-up vest. The surgeon and two on-looking students laughed in surprise at my readiness.

§

One week after surgery. The evening before my second post-op appointment, with a very serious look, my mom handed me the phone. "Your surgeon."

What a surprise. A call. And just twelve hours before my appointment. I didn't connect the dots. "Hi!"

Chapter 22

Mom studied my face while I listened to my surgeon. "During surgery, the two lymph nodes taken were tested, and came back negative." (That's good.) "Then, they were sent off, frozen, and cut at different angles for further testing. They came back positive." (You don't want to hear that.) "This happens in only 2% of the population. I've scheduled surgery two weeks out—October 26—to remove all lymph nodes from both your arms. Or, you can wait three to four months until your implant surgery. We either need to do it right away, or wait until the scars heal. Think about it and come with your answer tomorrow."

I hung up the phone, looked at my mom across the room and said, "I need to call Marilyn." (The minister I'd been leaning into for counseling.)

The following day, my mom drove me to the clinic and sat in on the appointment. The doctor suggested removal of all lymph nodes from both arms, radiation everyday for six weeks, and five years of medication, Tamoxifen or Arimidex. Relatively quickly we removed radiation from the list. She felt I would benefit from all treatments, but said the other two were much higher on her list for me, and in combination would work well, while preserving the aesthetics of my reconstruction. She gave me percentages of reoccurrence if I proceeded with all suggested treatment. Then, percentages with each treatment on its own, various combinations, or doing no further treatment at all. I told her I still didn't have an answer for her. It was Thursday. She told me to call the office Monday with an answer regarding surgery the following week.

We shifted our attention to my drains. They were pulled out. I immediately had more mobility. Hooray! My surgeon watched as the student doctor pulled the first drain from one side of my ribcage. I asked him to warn me before he pulled so I could fully exhale to reduce any pain.

He honored that. "Ready?"

I exhaled. He yanked the tube. Like receiving a sudden slack in a tug-of-war rope, his arms flailed to catch his balance when my body released the tube. It shocked both of us, his hand careening into my breast—two weeks after surgery.

§

Within an hour of my mom and I getting home, my friend Mike, from Los Angeles, was at the door. We talked very little about the choices I'd just been given. We laughed a lot in spite of such heavy, unexpected news.

He left the next afternoon. My mom drove fifty miles north to my place again, staying the night on the air mattress that never seemed to get inflated enough. While she was driving to my place, Mom's "check battery" light flashed on in her car. She doesn't know the layout of my city, so the following morning, together we took her car in for a battery. While the mechanic swapped batteries, I didn't budge from the passenger seat. Mom sat in the back, reading the paper. I slept off and on. I hurt. I felt miserable.

We got home and before Mom left, Carol, my next "on duty" friend arrived. She was the first person to stay five hours instead of overnight. At the "changing of the guards" I had a hissy fit. I'd had no time at all for myself, and two helpers in front of me at once—but no one lined up for the following week. Through tears of frustration and fatigue I shared, "I haven't even had time alone to poop! I know I need people here. I appreciate everyone helping me. I'm just scared—mostly over food preparation for next week." Carol arrived with a pile of magazines to read, expecting me to sleep. (I had told her that's what I did.) She ended up cooking almost the entire time while I slept, overloaded, hurting and stressed out.

For the next few days I wept off and on. I felt the weight of the world on me: What the medical field was suggesting, versus what I felt I should do. I was aware that I was scared, and that I was ignorant and in denial when my journey with cancer began. My desire was to walk away from the medical suggestions, but I was aware that might not serve me well.

§

After-surgery recovery included no driving for four weeks. My counseling sessions were on the phone for that month. The first week I cried through most of the hour-long session. Feelings ranged from fear to sorrow for what I had dragged my mom and Mary through. I could see they were tired, and they still showed up to help me. I had been at my worst with them—moody, demanding, weak, and dependent. My fear not only stemmed from medical decisions I needed to make, but from whether I'd made the right decision with having implants versus prosthetics. I had expanders now, and experienced pain with them—again, as with the port placement, because I'm thin. My "new friends," the expanders, didn't have added padding provided from body fat in which to snuggle.

Also pulling me down: Too much time to think. I'd wonder what input John would've had on all this—and how he'd respond. We'd each been through our own life-changing experience this year without correspondence with each other. He moved from one extremely remote area in Afghanistan to another. Because he was living as a nomad, there was no address. Until five months into his six-month deployment, I heard from him only once a month, when he arrived at an area having Internet access (and long lines of others waiting their turn). After a shower, good meal, and a day to repack, he'd head out again. I was head-over-heels for this man. It had been ten months since he left for a six-month duty. It was October, and I hadn't received an email since May 22. I leaned into knowing we both had strong faith, and a sense we were a match for each other. This was my time to heal. I had an intense feeling that when he came home, things would move fast.

§

Monday afternoon, October 19. I thought it over. I prayed. I meditated. Sought counseling from a minister, and my intern psychologist. I was at peace with my decision. I called the surgeon's office and canceled the surgery scheduled for October 26. My main reason was quality of life. Out of twenty to thirty lymph nodes, I only had two removed. This resulted in limiting my range of motion. I had (and have) numbness under my arm where the lymph nodes were taken.

If I were to have all of my lymph nodes removed, there would be seemingly endless precautions for infection prevention. I opted to live in the now. Fully. One precaution really got my attention: Even a thorn prick from a rose could start an infection. I've been told, "Don't go barefoot." "Be very cautious with hot objects—including sun or steam. Jacuzzi use isn't recommended." "Use extra care with sharp things—things with sharp edges." I've been so cavalier with Saltine crackers! "Wear a compression sleeve while stressing the affected arm." That meant repetitive motion of exercise, or household chores; being in high altitudes, or lifting something heavy. Gardening and air travel—two of my favorites, came with big warnings.

§

After I'd had a pretty low week, Mom came up and we had a blast! She brought everything with her to make Pepparkakor. It's a traditional Swedish cookie similar to a gingerbread cookie. I watched her do the work from across the counter. We shared childhood memories we each had. Then she said, "You have wonderful people in your life. Many people ask about you, pray for you, and love you." I knew it, but hearing it brought things into perspective.

Chapter 22

A friend I hadn't seen in over a year came up for several hours. I didn't have loads for her to do, but appreciated her ironing a shirt and completing my to-do list. I hesitated asking her to help, but she kept coming to mind, so I called her. Her daughter had had cancer, and died halfway through chemo a few years ago. My friend kept telling me how glad she was I allowed her to help. I am so blessed to have the friends and family I do!

§

I live a five-minute walk from a lagoon. I walked down the steep driveway to the benches, and sat down. Then, I walked up the slope and rested at the top—standing, hunched over with my hands on my hips, panting. When I caught my breath I walked back down the hill and repeated the process three times. It was the longest, and most strenuous walk I'd done in four months. I came home wiped out, but proud of my new endurance level. At 5:30 p.m., exhausted, I staggered to bed and slept until 8:30 a.m.. I awoke sneezing, with a cold, and used Kleenex all day. The immune system is so fragile.

E-mail Updates

Dear Natalie,

Thanks again to you, and Allison. I've been eating nonstop since!

—Allison: Picked a pack of perfect peaches for a patient perfectly pleased.

—Cherisse: Claudia cheered while chowing Cherisse's cooked chicken cake encased with incredible crust!

—Natalie: Knowingly kneads her nurturing nature numerous ways into noteworthy neurons.

happy weekend to you!

Love,

Claudia

§

Thanks for the rhymes Claudia!!! You are so creative! It sure felt strange not to give you a hug yesterday, I'll have to get two next week! If you want to chat or if you need anything, here is my cell number. I think you might already have it, but I wanted to make sure.

I was thinking about our conversation yesterday — whether you are scared or strong. I suppose it's not really my place to be telling you what you are, but through my eyes, you are brave. You are scared (because we all would be) but you are moving forward — one foot in front of the other every single day and that makes you brave. If you weren't scared, you wouldn't have the opportunity to be brave. And that bravery is yours forever. You are moving through all of this emotionally and physically. It's messy, but it should be, you are human and you are brave.

Best,

Natalie

§

Dear Karen,

To answer your question about if I sleep well. I seem to do "4-hour shifts," waking up when pain meds wear off.

I also take heavy pain meds for the expanders, which are empty. I had no idea they'd hurt, and man do they! Now I have a fear of going in every week (once I get the nerve to start) to expand the skin. Millions of women do it by choice, so I can, too! (The good news is I don't want to be

Chapter 22

bigger than I was, and they say, almost laughing at me, that won't take long. The only photos they've shown me are of big bodied, big busted women.) As with the port, I do not have fat for the foreign object to nestle under, so I feel it. I honestly think I'm the smallest breasted woman they've dealt with. How strange . . . 34B?

I'm not driving due to the heavy meds. It's a bit like being under house arrest, I suppose.

Nothing but cheer from this side of the street!

Hope your side is brighter, and known as Easy Street! I'll be there soon.

Love,

C

§

Dear Allan,

I thought of you this morning. For the third time in the last few months (you better sit down) . . . I've had a bean sandwich! (the first time I had it cold on white bread, cheese on top). Now, I toast wheat bread, warm up the beans and add cheese. It's not exactly a meal I'd have done if I had loads of energy, but it's one of the first meals I've made on my own.

I've canceled the Oct 26 surgery, and am waiting for surgeon to call me to answer more questions. I seem to keep asking questions they answer, "We don't know." I told my Dad about the latest news. He was in such shock—which brought me to tears—that he had handed the phone to his wife to have me tell her what the doctor said. His wife urged, "You've GOT to listen to them." I told her I'd make the right decision for me at the right time.

Anyway, my new boobs hurt—the expander is under the muscle—which is new territory. Ouch. When I wake up it feels really tight, like rope friction around my chest. Once I get moving, it's OK. I keep getting a sensation like goose bumps, but don't see any. The nerves were cut, and are scrambled. I wonder if it's sort of like phantom pain. My underarm (where lymph nodes were taken) hurts like hell. I asked if it will hurt more than it does now if they take out all lymph nodes, they don't know. Everything seems SO individual.

Love,

Claudia

§

Look, whatever state you are in, trust me, a cold baked bean sandwich on white bread, with loads of butter is a tonic. Doctors here issue prescriptions for baked beans (along with marmite—not to be combined) AND it's a perfect balance of protein, carbs, etc. So don't you poo poo it as some inferior snack that you have in place of a meal!

I'm not surprised you cancelled the surgery and don't be concerned about asking lots of questions. That's the way to go even if they struggle with the answer. What do you mean your new boobs? I thought you didn't have new boobs yet. Bugger about the pain—there will come the day soon when you are pain free. Yes, one of the problems is that a lot of this is so individual. And it's also done on percentages. I actually agree that you've GOT to listen to them. It doesn't mean you don't make your own decision. You still have to weigh up the options and the effect on your life. Just don't forget

Chapter 22

that even allowing for some restrictions/limitations, your obligation to yourself and everyone else is to live!

Oh dear this is getting too deep so better sign off and talk to you this weekend.

Take care,

Allan

§

Dear Allan,

I told a friend about the baked bean meal, and she said, "That's a guy's meal." Why does everyone else know about this meal and not me? Hmmm . . . yes, I did blow it off as inferior. Silly me.

Next week I have an appointment with the surgeon, the oncologist, and the following week with a neurologist. Still haven't made first appointment to begin filling the expanders. Now they tell me expanders may hurt the whole way through—yikes. Don't have much wiggle room for skin to stretch. I feel every bit of it.

As for not having girly shape yet, it's better than I thought. I expected craters from the removal. I was pleasantly surprised to find I had some shape left and now understand when they kept saying how small my breasts were, they were talking about the breast tissue. (So, I'm probably a size smaller on one side, and two sizes smaller on the other side.)

I just reread the last part of your email. Wow. That is deep. Yikes. I missed it first time around. My Dad was really shaken up when I told him what was going on (after we'd had a long, general conversation, he said, "Anything else going on?"—"Uh, actually, yes . . . .") He then called every few days. I finally told him, "I'm *not dying, and it's my decision." He's backed off his calling to once a week and really dances around* . . . . *"Sooooo . . . any doctor appointments this week???" Oh well. Nice to be loved.*

Take care,

Love,

C

§

Just a quick note to say oh my goodness, I cant believe I got away with the 'deep' bits. First thing I've done since I got home was check my e-mail cos I was expecting to get such a slap for giving advice. Whew. Thought it would amuse you to know that you kept me on edge for a while. I'll do a proper e-mail on the weekend or give you a call.

Cheers for now,

Allan

§

Dear Cathy,

Walked to the lagoon again today. I left the house in wool socks, fleece pants, wool long underwear top, silk scarf, and wind resistant fleece jacket. After the first hill, I realized it was warmer outside than I thought. Came home and shifted to short sleeve top, lighter socks, no jacket—then got cold, sneezed over 50 times in an hour, so I'm back to (lighter) wool socks, and lighter pants, and top! Jacket and scarf is nearby if I go outside.

And people ask me what I do during the day?!

Have a good one!

Chapter 22

Love you,

Claudia

§

Dear Mike,

You've been on my mind, and I thank you for your willingness to grow in order to support me this year. It's meant tons to me.

Took off the bandages last night—glad you saw it when you did. It looked scary to me. Everything looks scary this week. I've had an hour of meltdowns this morning as I've been getting ready to go to Dr appt. I was all dressed up, then put on shoes and could not walk across the room because of neuropathy pain in my feet. Tried different shoes several times before getting into jeans and tennis shoes—a real big let down. Would like to get out of jeans, yoga pants.

Today I'm joining an eight-week support group that's also a research study group. My surgeon got me into in it. Maybe it was my attitude and comment this week about lymph node removal. "Having had cancer, I guess I'm uninsurable. Is that why you want to take everything out now?" blah blah blah—

Love,

Claudia

Tips for Him or Her:

✔ Get a pack of Dentswab (those little sponge lollipops). They're great for the dry mouth you'll have after surgeries.

✔ Constipated? Have I got tricks for you! And you'll need them, especially after any surgery. Make a fist. Rub your stomach in a clockwise motion, down on the left, up on the right. (Now pat your head. Just joking.) Slowly make a circular motion five to ten times with your fist. I took an extra-strength stool softener four times a day the first few days after surgery. (They can also be taken after chemo treatments if needed.) Also, a few minutes of walking, or other activity helps. Good and Plenty candy (or black licorice in any form) works, too. Fluids: Tea, water, juice. Drink plenty of them. It isn't about drinking lots at once, it's about staying hydrated. For me, twenty-four to forty-eight hours after surgery, almost everything was too acidic. Hot water and honey, tea, or watered down, warm prune juice were comforting. Be patient. It may take five to six days for things to get moving again. Keep the fluids and reasonable amounts of fiber going in.

✔ Get your information from your medical team rather than searching the Internet. If you want to gather additional information call the American Cancer Society at (800) 227-2345 or consult reputable websites like www.cancer.gov (the American Cancer Society's website) and www.breastcancer.org.

Tips for Those Who Want to Help:

✔ Don't know what to do? Ask. But look around and think for yourself first. Conserve their energy. Ask them, "What would help you?" "What would you like?" "Would you like [a drink of water]? Or, "I noticed you were out of [xyz]—would you like me to pick more up?"

✔ Offer a hospital or home visit.

Chapter 22

✔ Create a basket for them. Or skip the basket and bring over things like: fruit, Fiber One bars, bran muffins, prunes, prune juice, or a water bottle or two.

✔ A neighbor made muffins for me after surgery. I loved them. Now I keep them on hand in the freezer, and make them for friends in need. I buy Bob's Red Mill Whole Ground Flaxseed Meal. The recipe is on the back of the bag. To your health!

Chapter 23

AFTER THE EARTHQUAKE

Neurontin, also known as Gabapentin, is a medication for neuropathy—numbness and pain usually in the hands and feet. As a side effect of Taxol, the drug I was given during the second round of chemo, I had neuropathy. The medication is the same one used for people coming off long-term marijuana use. Gabapentin has a great side benefit of helping decrease hot flashes, but an annoying drawback of causing dizziness and blurred vision. My fingers had that slammed-in-a-drawer feeling. I couldn't button small buttons, and the tips of my fingers buzzed. My feet had an ice-burning sensation of thawing. Each step felt like fire walking on golf balls.

My gait changed as a result of neuropathy. Getting out of a chair or car became quite an ordeal. I decided it was unacceptable. I joined the Boys and Girls Club, and the women in the pool there for an arthritis exercise class. We slowly moved our legs and arms for one hour. On my first day I came home and dove for the couch to sleep for an hour. I was in bed by 7 p.m. for twelve hours of hibernation. I had to pace myself. If I gave it a "decent" workout, I was too exhausted to go to class the next day. If I had anything else planned that day, I skipped the pool. The few times I pushed it, I caught a cold. It just wasn't worth it.

§

I called the American Cancer Society and asked them to connect me with women my age who'd had a mastectomy and a sentinel node dissection, and who either took or had taken Tamoxifen or Arimidex. I'd done my research; now I wanted to talk with others to see what they had to say. I was connected with four women, two near my age. These wonderful women each contacted me and shared their stories, helping me make a clear decision about taking Tamoxifen, Arimidex, or neither.

From these calls, I learned many women stop the reconstruction process for various reasons. Some have just had it with being poked and prodded, and are ready to get on with life. One woman told me she walked away at the nipple stage. Another shared that she waited ten years before going back for an implant. She acknowledged the expanders were painful, but encouraged me to keep moving forward now if I could stand it.

§

I attended another support group, primarily to hear if anyone was taking Arimidex, and if not, why? This group was a research study group where everyone committed to eight weekly meetings. The group consisted of six women. I was the oldest at forty-four, the only one not married, and the only one with expanders. Three of the six had very large breasts. (Two naturally large, one with wildly large implants for her body.) In her introduction, she shared with excitement, "They're so much larger than they've ever been!" (I could guess that!) These same three women were very talkative. Even while I introduced myself, they jumped in, asking me questions. It got very quiet when I answered, "No" to questions about my having further surgery, radiation, and taking Tamoxifen or Arimidex. Everyone else in this group was doing everything their doctors suggested. All of them had support at home, and one

Chapter 23

of them had to be reminded by the facilitator that chemo wasn't the breeze for her that she now reminisced.

One woman had just been diagnosed that week. She shared her desire for a bilateral mastectomy, not even knowing she needed a mastectomy of any sort. (A week after my diagnosis my head spun for ways to prove there'd been a mistake!) Proof that everyone goes through this in their own way.

I didn't connect with the women in this group. The next day I called the facilitator, apologizing for not sticking to the agreement. "I'm calling to inform you I'm quitting the group. I get so much more out of my one-to-one counseling sessions. I feel I'm moving forward there, not looking back."

I hung up the phone and sent my counselor for the one-to-one sessions a thank you card. At our next session, I brought her a "diamond." In recent past, she used the diamond as an analogy for the person I've become. She sent me this, which she found on the Internet:

Diamonds are incredibly sought after and valued not only for their beauty, but because they are the hardest natural substance. As we go through life, we are exposed to a variety of trials and just as the carbon, we are susceptible to the pressures and heat that trials may bring. Through the process, there may be times where the pressure and heat becomes unbearable, and we may question our ability to continue. During these times it is often difficult to see beyond the immediate present, but if we develop the capacity to view our potential, we gain the perspective that after the trial we have become just like the diamond, strong, beautiful, and of infinite worth.

§

My counselor also used the analogy of cancer being an earthquake. My entire foundation was shaken. Then, I stood in distress amongst the rubble. Next came the rebuilding. She reminded me that after rebuilding the foundation, I'd get to choose whatever I wanted. I really connected with the earthquake analogy.

It made me think of a beautiful sculpture in Napier, New Zealand. *The Spirit of Napier,* by Frank Szirmay, was created in memory of the 1931 earthquake that flattened the town. Now, a bronze, nude woman stands on a concrete pillar, her arms reaching upward, showing she's risen from the hard times of the earthquake.

Cancer is like an earthquake. And each individual can rise from the rubble and debris caused by that earthquake. I was reminded: I am persistent, resilient, and good at honing-in on inner strength and working my way through various situations. You can, too!

E-mail Updates

> *Dear Michele,*
>
> *I think of you often. You've been a shining light for me, and I know my journey is temporary. I hope the fatigue and mood swings are too . . . .*
>
> *The woman I see for counseling put it this way yesterday, "It's like an earthquake—it shakes the entire foundation." And now I'm rebuilding. That's a great analogy for me.*
>
> *Love you,*
>
> *C*

§

yes

i know

it shook you

and not in a good pina colada way

and definitely the meds and lack of good nutrition

add to that

i know you are rebuilding

Chapter 23

be gentle with yourself

i love you

it's all good

Michele

§

Dear Marion,

Do you remember way back when . . . . You gave me fruit, offered to pick up things from the store for me, took me to the store—and cut the watermelon when we got home, prepared a festive welcome back, and taught me Callanetics? I remember way back when . . . . You're one of the blessings for whom I'm grateful. THANKS FOR GIVING

~Claudia~

§

Thank you Claudia,

This has brought tears to my eyes, you are a very special person. That's why you are in the business you're in, I know!!

§

Dear Michele,

For carrying me through your e-mails. I give thanks.

For the cards you sent and the love in them. I give thanks.

For making me laugh, and allowing me to get way too serious, deep, dark and pitiful. I give thanks. For calling me before I went into surgery. I give thanks.

For holding to the vision I will get to Florida and see you!!! I give thanks.

You are one of the blessings for whom I'm grateful.

Much love,

Claudia

§

girlfriend . . . i accept, with one exception

you are never pitiful . . . never ever

I'm thankful, you took a liking to a clown

I'm thankful that through you i know fancy nancy

I'm thankful you'll be floating in my pool

and teaching me more than you already have

you are the most honest person i know

hugs,

Michele

Tips for Him or Her:

✔ Do your post-mastectomy exercises, and others to reduce or prevent lymphedema. Practice raising your arms over your head while keeping your elbows straight. Later, you might use 12-16 ounce cans of food, or water bottles as weights, moving up to the liter size (2.2 pounds). Gradually, you'll move to 5-pound weights. Everyday activities will build your strength, too.

✔ You can pick up trash on walks as part community good, part exercise. I did this too soon. I later did it once a week. Give yourself time to work up to it. I was soooo stiff and sore afterward! Wear gloves, or use one of those trash grabbers.

✔ Have someone go grocery shopping with you to do the heavy lifting.

✔ If you're traveling before you have strength back, consider shipping a box to your destination instead of hauling luggage. For a trip from California to Florida, then Arkansas, I ground shipped a box to Arkansas a few days before I left. It cost me the same as checking the bag with the airlines, but saved me the hassle. Figure $1.00 per pound. Take a lightweight carry on.

✔ Revise your expectations for recovery time. Allow yourself to adjust to the changes from cancer. Some women can jump right back into their pre-cancer activities, or walk for cancer fundraisers the following week. Treatments vary, and so does recovery time. Honor your body.

Chapter 24

REBUILDING BARBIE

November. Okay, sit down for this one . . . . My nose hair was coming back! Ha! So were my eyelashes, and yes, my not-so-public hair, too. Whoopee! The doctor thinks a gap in my eyebrow will fill in, and says my eyelashes will lengthen. (I had long, lush lashes, and now they're short and sparse.)

§

At my December oncology appointment I demanded an answer. "I've been out of chemo three months. My hair is coming back on my head. Why don't I have energy to do things?"

The doctor looked at me straight on and said, "You have been through major treatment, followed by major surgery. This is big stuff. Your body's healing."

"Oh."

"Give yourself one to two years to recover."

I wasn't sure when energy and strength would come roaring back. The lack of vitality brought me down for so long. I felt my quality of life had been stripped away. Then, I'd remind myself, it's all perspective, and that I was blessed.

I arrived for my first scheduled expansion appointment scared. I felt I wasn't getting the information I needed. Through tears I said,

"I still hurt from surgery. I need to know more about this process before I do it. I'm not ready to start yet."

I'd seen a full-size expander, a disk-shaped plastic balloon that expands when saline is injected into it, thus stretching my skin. But I had a half-size kidney-shaped expander. I'd already seen an implant, but seeing a 500 cc implant when I'll have a 200 cc implant was a shock, and fed my fear of having implants larger than I wanted.

The medical assistant said, "Some women are more sensitive and hurt longer after surgery. Reschedule two weeks out. We'll start with 40 cc of saline instead of 60 cc."

Just about skipping out of the office, I knew I'd made the right decision! I came back two weeks later, ready to start the process.

§

Beginning the breast expansion process for reconstruction, once again I was told how small my breasts were. I finally said, "It's not like I bought my 34B bras at a specialty store." I had expanders in that held 200 cc of saline (about 20 tablespoons).

The medical assistant said, "Most women with a 200 cc expander fill it at 60-120 cc at a time. They're done in two-to-four visits."

I asked, "Why do some women say the expansion process is excruciating?"

Without much attention, she replied, "Could be from filling the expanders too quickly."

Note to self: Don't do 60 cc on my first visit!

The process: The site was sterilized with alcohol wipes, then with a little magnet they found the port (the dark center in the expander). They marked the spot with a felt tip pen so they would know where to put the syringe needle to inject the saline. I sat and waited for about ten minutes before the injection while anesthetic

Chapter 24

cream numbed the site. I could feel the expander stretching my skin when it reached about 25 cc. My skin got tight around 30 cc.

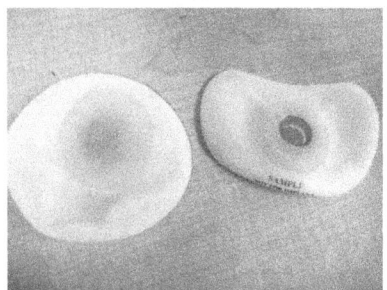

Types of expanders - I had the half size

Several months after the expansion, the implants are placed, then the cherries on top (AKA nipples). When they first told me that, I felt woozy (only to learn much later the idea of having to wait for nipples wasn't nearly as "wooze-inducing" as hearing from where they get the nipple skin! Pull up a chair. Oh, on second thought, maybe not! Best to stay standing!).

§

"Do you have any tattoos?" That was one of John's first questions. I said, "No." That was then . . . . But now he had been in Afghanistan for just under a year, and around that time I learned that several months after getting cherries in place, they would tattoo the areola on! Oh my goodness! At exactly what point would the knees stop knocking? When the hell would the shock waves stop? I kept thinking I knew what was coming—then I'd get more knee-buckling news. Couldn't I just hear I'd won the lotto, or something like that?

Now when someone asked if I had any tattoos, I guess I'd say, "Yes."

Of course, they would follow with, "How many?"

"One."

"Where?"

I supposed I'd tell them, "My breast."

You can see the reaction: Raised eyebrows (providing they aren't in chemo, lacking eyebrows). A slow broadening grin which begged the questions: "Of what? "Can I see?"

E-mail Updates

Happy belated birthday! I hope you had a wonderful day yesterday!

Today I thank God for your next year and for bringing you through the last one.

Claudia, I also want to thank you for coming to the class on Saturday and for the donation to Heifer International. You know, we may have fed you here and there, but you fed us too and I'm so grateful for you. You inspire me. In your strength, in your weakness, in your victories and in your struggles—you inspire me. Thank you so much for coming to the class and supporting me. It meant so much to me to have you there. You are a peaceful presence for me and it was wonderful to see you.

Enjoy your day! Today, tomorrow, and onward!

Love,

Natalie

§

Missed your birthday, as usual, sigh. Why are you wearing a scarf? You look great. Maybe the hair is a bit shorter than current US fashion, I don't know, but who cares. Be a trendsetter. I will give you a call soon. Only 2 days of work to go and then I can relax.

Cheers for now, Allan

Chapter 24

§

Dear Allan,

No worries about the b-day. I took the package you sent as birthday/Christmas anyway. The NZ ornaments you sent are the only decorations I have out this year. My favorites are the angel and the Maori meetinghouse. Stayed at Mom's for my b-day for two days. As soon as I got there (an hour drive) I took a nap, then off to the dentist for a cleaning. They were thrilled I "only" have one cavity. HUH?! They said usually after chemo, they see a mouth full of cavities due to dry mouth. After a snooze, my cousin and one of Mom's previous neighbors came over and we had fish tacos.

Not one person mentioned anything about cancer. I saw my sister the next day, and one of my brothers called Mom's after I'd left. No one mentioned it. I came home and was exhausted. It was the furthest I'd driven since Easter. I came home and cried about how no one seemed to "get it." Then realized, again, it is my journey, and no one else can "get it." Although some have come close, and you are one of those. Thanks.

I wear a scarf because it's cold without it (it's winter in So Cal, you know). When I get hot flashes, I take it off—and eat Otter Pops! I also take off the scarf when I'm in the pool! I had to buy a comb. I was starting to look like a little kid who's been out playing hard. Really, with scarf, I find people are very nice, letting me in front of the line etc. I recently had to stand longer than I'd planned while I waited for Kinko's to print out a booklet I made Mom. (Top 100 reasons why I love you—not in order; not all inclusive.) I didn't want to just give Mom 4 separate pages, or I'd have done it on my own. Lucky chance—the store had a chair on display nearby! I grabbed it, moved it over to the counter and sat while the lady made the booklet. I think people would've raised an eyebrow (I love that phrase now that I have them back!) had they not seen a scarf.

My Dad was interviewed for his local newspaper and sent me the newspaper article only after several of his friends and neighbors suggested he send the article to his kids. It gave me info I didn't know about his career. You may find it interesting. If you want, I'll copy it and send it to you. Have you read the book I sent you yet? (Fire From The Sky).

Take Care,

Love

C

§

Firstly, the journey. I haven't figured it totally but there are reasons people don't mention it, and I don't think it is because they are uncaring. The bottom line is that people just don't get it. Unless they know you really well, (and sometimes even more so then) people will be hesitant. If they encounter you looking happy, enjoying yourself they'll think, oh I won't spoil it by mentioning that. Or simply, should I mention that, should I ask, etc. I could go on but essentially people aren't confident/comfortable dealing with this kinda stuff. And it scares people. Talk more about this.

Good points re the scarf. Forgot how cold it gets over there! Yes you do need a signal at times that tells people there's something going on here, I'm not just a lazy ass. Kinkos? Sounds like some sort of sex club for perverts.

What the hell are Otter Pops?

Chapter 24

Love to read the article—no, not read the book yet. My time for reading soon.

Only tomorrow to go then off work, yay.

Cheers,

Allan

Tips for Him or Her:

✔ The idea behind expanders is to stretch the skin. Not everyone who has expanders experiences pain. If you still hurt from surgery when your first expansion is scheduled, reschedule. Ask them to fill you less on each visit, or every other week instead of weekly. Also, ibuprofen for a few days after each fill, and perhaps even prescription strength pain reliever for the day of expansion. Thin women seem to have more expander-related pain than other women.

✔ There are some great options to help fade scars. An aesthetic-conscious plastic surgeon does wonders. So does emu oil. And many scars fade over time. To speed up the process, Mederma gel, www.mederma.com or ScarLine Rx, www.scarline.com may help. ScarLine Rx is a medical-grade silicone that comes in various shapes and sizes for any raised or red scars. It's worn for twelve hours a day, for at least ninety days.

✔ Get a temporary disabled parking permit if you need one. This was really helpful the first few months I was driving again, especially when neuropathy was affecting my walking. It saved me from using my energy in the parking lot. Google "DMV temporary disabled parking," choose your state (geographic, not emotional), complete your portion of the form, and have your doctor complete his or her portion. Then send in your money. Don't abuse this privilege.

Chapter 25

LYMPHEDEMA: JUST THE FACTS, MA'AM

While still in the gathering-information stage about lymphedema, this is what I learned:

Even though I had a sentinel node dissection, with only two lymph nodes removed, it was highly suggested I get a compression sleeve and gauntlet as a precaution for flying. There's concern of infection and arm swelling due to the lymphatic system's not being able to work as well after any lymph nodes are taken. It can take a month for lymphedema swelling to decrease, and there's lots of hassle that goes with it—having the limb wrapped and immobilized, and the aesthetics of the limb swelling to three times its original size.

A hospital (not mine) had grant money not used, and awarded me a full grant for my first two compression sleeves and gauntlets. What a gift!

The sleeve should be worn for exercising, gardening, walks/hikes, high altitudes, or repetitive motions like sweeping and scrubbing. A reason to get a maid! Not wearing the sleeve and gauntlet (or glove) is a huge risk when stressing the arm from which the lymph nodes were taken. This stuff scared me. I'm part ostrich (head in the sand), or, as I prefer to think—an optimist (head in the clouds). I had been sleeping lots at this point. I think it may have been a bit of depression. All these precautions sounded like one more dig at freedom.

Some days I could get my rings on, but without much wiggle room, so I didn't wear them. I learned how to do my own lymph drainage massage. Some people like to use a dry brush on their skin. I found it too harsh and didn't want another "ball and chain" to pack everywhere I went. I used my hand instead.

Cancer put a bit of a dark cloud on the happy-go-lucky life. I seldom walked the beach barefoot anymore, and no longer went barefoot on the sidewalk—just too many new dangers. I looked at Jacuzzis in a new way, too. Red wine is also on the precaution list for lymphedema. During this time the voice of caution rattled loudly in my head. It was a big disappointment, but you move forward the best you can, and keep wisdom close at hand. On the bright side, I heard a recent change to the red wine rule. It's not about avoiding the occasional drink of alcohol or soda, but to drink equal part of water before or after.

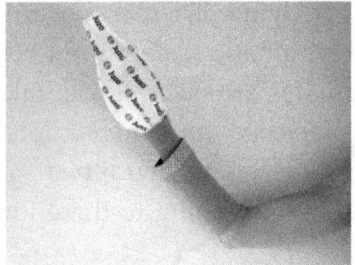
Compressing the sleeve half way on

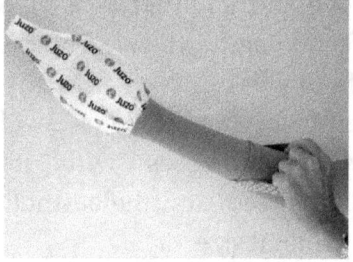
Pulling the sleeve up

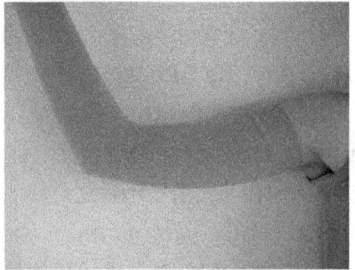
Positioning the sleeve

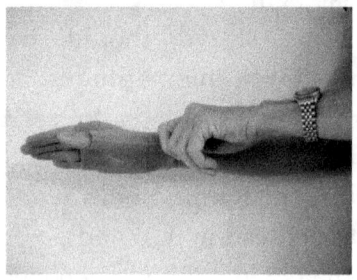
Gauntlet, overlapping sleeve

Chapter 25

Tips for Him or Her:

✔ Go to the official Lymphology Association of North America (LANA) website, www.clt-lana.org, and search the list of Certified LANA Therapists.

✔ Get measured for compression garments. If you require one custom made, it could add $50.00 to the cost, but proper fit is crucial. Insurance doesn't cover the garment, and they need replacing every six months, if used frequently. They're about $100.00-$200.00 for each piece.

✔ Wear your compression sleeve as a precaution, and anytime your hand or arm feels heavy, numb or tingly. Also, anytime you're stressing the lymphatic system: Lifting weights at the gym, traveling in high altitudes, or doing repetitive activities like kayaking, or chores like mopping. When flying, reach up frequently. I haven't used deodorant since surgery—I claim I don't need it. I'll have to test my theory on a flight.

✔ How to put on the extremely snug compression sleeve: Roll the top part of the sleeve almost halfway down the original length, and inside-out so the silicone bumps are showing. Flatten the wrinkles. Cup your hand and push through the wide end while using your other hand to help pull up the sleeve (don't use fingernails!). To help stabilize your arm, use a wall, or your car if you're heading into the gym. Once the narrow end of the sleeve is at your wrist, flatten any wrinkles and continue pulling up the folded half. When you're done, the silicone should be against your skin, close to your axilla. If there's a seam, it should run on the outside of the arm near the elbow.

✔ Another option for donning the sleeve with relative ease is to spread a pinch of corn starch over the arm. Be positive your arm is dry, or it'll be a muddy mess. A compression sleeve Slippie is a slick, Tyvek cone that fits over the hand and arm. Your LANA therapist may have an extra Slippie, especially if you've purchased your garment from them. Otherwise, search online. The sleeve glides!

✔ A dishwashing glove worn on the opposite hand can help inch-up the sleeve.

✔ Do not wear a compression garment while sleeping, or one garment without the other.

✔ Keep moisturized. It prevents breakdown of the skin—a big deal with lymphedema. Allow ten to fifteen minutes for lotion to absorb before wearing a garment. Lotion and oil shorten the garment's life. If you oil, do it at night or when you know you won't be wearing the sleeve.

✔ Avoid tight clothing, or jewelry becoming tight on the affected limb. You may want to wear bracelets instead of rings. If your hand swells, a ring could be dangerous.

✔ Know your body so you're aware if you need to make changes to your routine, or if you need medical attention.

✔ Static bouncing (sitting on a balance ball or jogging on a small trampoline), swimming, or scuba diving are all fantastic for the lymphatic system! These activities help prevent and reduce early stage lymphedema. Grab an exercise balance ball, sit on it—and bounce for about ten minutes. You may feel a post nasal drip, or the need to clear your throat.

✔ Do not allow anyone to take your blood pressure or use needles on the arm from which lymph nodes have been taken. Some suggest a medical alert bracelet, and while in the hospital, use colored, painter's masking tape on the affected arm, and write on the tape: "DO NOT USE NEEDLES OR TAKE BLOOD PRESSURE ON THIS ARM." (This tip from a woman who was in the hospital, and the big, neon cardboard sign at the head of her bed didn't work. She'd awake to find staff and a blood pressure cuff on her affected arm. Her father showed up with the colored masking tape. Communication cleared up.)

Chapter 25

✔ Learn lymph drainage massage. As you follow your individualized body map given to you by your therapist, use the same weight of your hand that you would for petting a big dog. I can feel the drainage happen relatively quickly. My hand tingles, I get a post nasal drip type response, and need to clear my throat. I'd strongly recommend learning lymph drainage by finding a certified lymphedema therapist. With lymphedema, smaller, slow strokes are best, rather than the long, typical massage type stroke.

Chapter 26

MAN MADE—NEVER "FAKE"

A Year Later

January. The appointment with my reconstruction surgeon didn't go smoothly. I thought we were going to talk about sizes and styles of implants. He was visibly upset when I pointed to my breasts and said, "Between this size, or the last expansion size."

He had expected, "This is exactly what I want." I freaked out over the aesthetics of the expanders—which I'd been told were not for aesthetics, but for the sole purpose of stretching the skin. I had a hard time seeing past the odd shape—especially without the top half, and one nipple. I told the surgeon I'd even gone searching online to look at reconstruction work, and was horrified at the sizes (huge) and shapes (grapefruit, watermelon, gourd). I couldn't relate to what I saw. He pointed to the mirror on the exam room door. "Look there! Are you saying you can't live with that?"

I stood there, looking, wiping away tears.

"You haven't come to terms with losing your breasts."

Who does? Does one ever?

He drew back his sharp arrow and let it fly, "This is not augmentation. This is reconstruction!"

Bull's eye! I burst into tears. He continued, "Go home and put on various tight fitting tops, put cotton on the top missing portion of your breast." (Skip this idea. Bumps of cotton made the whole attempt to see beauty impossible.) "Look in the mirror and come back and tell me the size you want. Frustrated, I yelled, "We are not communicating well today! I have nothing to compare! I have not studied naked women!"

Standing with hands on his hips, he kept asking, "What do you want?"

"34B to 34C maximum."

With temper ramping up, he said, "Don't tell me bra size. I can't work by bra size. Tell me what you want!" He gave me the example of shoe sizes. He said he's a 12.5 in one brand, and 13.5 in another brand. His point being that there's no standard for shoe or bra sizing.

I told him, "I'm going to Nordstrom to get measured." I could tell he thought that was dumb, which fueled my flame.

As we wound up (the appointment, not our arms to slug each other) he said, "I'm sorry I made you cry."

Full of pride, I wanted to say, *You didn't make me do anything.* Then, a not so small, or still voice came to my mind: *STOP!* I said, "I'm sorry—" Searching for a description, all I could quickly come up with was, "—for . . . for getting that way."

He blew it off, and handed me Kleenex.

I did go to Nordstrom to see a woman who has measured me over the years. I learned she specializes in sizing women who've had mastectomies. When I arrived, she was with a customer. Her coworker offered to help me. I explained why I was waiting, adding, "I hope I'm close to my previous 34B size." I got measured. In the singsong Nordstrom manner, she called out, "32D." I was shocked! Stunned! She confirmed the measurement then chirped, "You know, 32D is considered the perfect size."

As we walked out of the dressing room, her coworker said, "So, what's your size?"

Still shocked, I said, "32D!"

She responded, "Oh, you're so lucky!"

The woman who measured me grinned at her coworker, "Tell her your size."

Chapter 26

The woman rolled her eyes. "34B."
What a laugh.

§

On my way home, the reconstruction surgeon's comment, "This is not augmentation. This is reconstruction" haunted me. I realized this process is much different from a breast augmentation. Those women go in, and two hours later they've got the breasts they want. I went in every week, hurt like hell for one to three days, and still wish for what I had.

When I got home, I tried on all sorts of my tops and dresses, looking at the projection of my breasts and nothing else. Not shape. Not left versus right. Not placement. Purely projection.

§

Ab-so-lute-ly amazing! Nipple sparing! During surgery, they were able to spare one of my nipples. They cut around it. My own nipple is still intact. I'd heard they might take half of the nipple later, to build up the other side. I'd also heard—from two women who weren't in the medical profession, hadn't had breast cancer, and didn't know anyone who'd gone through this sort of reconstruction—tell me the skin for a new nipple comes from the vaginal area! WHAT? That is craaazy! The information came in such a casual manner with no regard to the topic being sensitive for the one hearing it, especially for the first time.

E-mail Updates

Dear Allan,

He [surgeon] is used to women who want to be big—I actually think he thinks I'm a bit of a freak, as I'm hung up on what I had, and he said I haven't gotten over the loss—and need to. Duh. I left the office yesterday mad, and in tears. They added four more tablespoons, and I freaked out, "This is way too big!!" They took a picture, showing this was max size. They need to stretch the skin beyond the size, so they can get the implant in, and close me up.

C

§

Stick to your guns over getting what you want. Why should you live with someone else's idea of how you should be, especially some bloke? You know best how you look, you don't want to be converted into how they think you should look. Sorry it's all so tough.

Be in touch over the next few days.

Cheers,

Allan

§

Dear Michele,

I just learned (via hearsay) that the skin to make new nipple is taken from vaginal area for color. Oh shit. I still can't believe it. I just never thought where it might come from! So, it's one more swipe at femininity and one more question I need answered: "Do I do this?" Right now I have one nipple, so either I need to add one, or give one back, or be OK with being "One-Eyed Betty." Will I be happy with that choice? It just makes my head spin. I had NO idea!

xo,

C

Chapter 26

§

OMG!!! such details . . . I say get a rose tattoo in place of the invisible nipple, keep the nipple you have, symmetry is highly overrated! I would say leave my Sissy ALONE. . . unless you are implanting something fun!

just my 2 cents.

Michele

February. My second post-chemo checkup appointment with my oncologist. Appointments will continue every three months for two years, every six-months for a year, then once a year. In September my oncologist strongly recommended my taking Tamoxifen or aromatase inhibitors daily for five years, minimum. Tamoxifen blocks estrogen receptive tumors from using estrogen. Aromatase inhibitors (Arimidex, Femara and Aromasin) reduce the body's amount of estrogen. Neither block ovary estrogen production, but aromatase inhibitors can block other tissues from making estrogen, which is why aromatase inhibitors only work in post-menopausal women. All these medications have similar side effects to chemo, but a lesser degree. I still had neuropathy, and wasn't in favor of more nausea, fatigue, and hair thinning, among other side effects. I told my oncologist, "I'll give it some thought and research, but I'm not leaning toward any more treatment, including medication . . . . If I said, 'No,' would you still retain me as your patient?"

"You'd have to do a lot worse than that! Yes, I'd keep you on as a patient, but I'll continue to recommend things such as Tamoxifen or aromatase inhibitors."

We both laughed. I said, "That's fine. My answer's 'no.'" I acknowledge him for his commitment to his views, and perhaps even more for his respecting—while not agreeing with—mine.

I also had an appointment with my reconstruction surgeon. His office was packed with people. He'd performed an emergency surgery in the morning and was running an hour behind schedule. As usual, I walked in with my pen and yellow note pad.

"This is the size I want," I told him.

He briefly squeezed, nudged, and eyed my breasts. "We'll leave this side alone and give two more expansions to the side with less skin. You'll be uneven for a few months but because more skin was taken, it's got to stretch more for the implant." In less then five minutes he was ready to leave the room.

Not so fast . . . . I reached for my list of questions.

"Could you walk me through the process of the nipple surgery? You mentioned you'd use part of the one spared, then build both sides up. Where does that skin come from?" Whooooa! I saw a deer meet headlights! I'm sure I returned the look.

His answer was a bullet point: "We're not there yet. Let's get through the implants first. There are three options, depending on each person's situation. It could come from behind the ear, the site itself, or the groin." (Interpretation: I have an office jam-packed with upset folks, and don't have the time for your meltdown now.) I felt optimistic about the term "groin" even if that was a safe, chicken-shit way of his dealing with me. It postponed further worry, and really, that's all I wanted.

I frequently needed pain medication for the first few days after an expansion, then ibuprofen for that week. Left over from my October surgery, I used Roxicodone, (oxycodone hydrochloride) which they said was too strong for my needs. "You're taking a gun to kill the fly on the wall." They wouldn't refill my prescription (Roxicodone is a narcotic).

I kept telling them, "I'm only taking it three days, every two weeks." The doctor prescribed Vicodin. It was like lying face-up on a fast spinning merry-go-round with my head toward the ground. The room spun, and at the same time I'd had a wild sensation of my

Chapter 26

feet being elevated above my head. I was wired and anxious. Needless to say, I never took it again. I told the doctor about it.

"I'll make a note that you have out-of-body experiences on Vicodin."

§

Mom and I attended a meeting for information on lymphedema. We met a woman who'd had surgery and no chemo. She said she was dancing again (a Scottish type of fast dance that takes loads of energy). Walking away from her, I cried. I came home and took two naps. Huh? I made it through chemo and surgery for this level of living? NO! I can't accept that.

Many would say, "If you're above ground, it's good." Hmmm . . . . The good news: My feet are feeling better—not as numb or painful.

§

March. I had a major meltdown over the whole breast implant thing. When I came up for air, I thought, how appropriate: "Seismic" refers to anything relating to an earthquake. I was feeling "size-mic pressures—not knowing what size! Implants would last for twelve to fifteen years. That felt like such a major commitment. I had heard stories where women told the doctor one size, and woke up being a much larger size. Some said, "Tell your doctor to implant a smaller size than what you want." I don't work like that. Honesty is where it is for me. In the midst of sobbing my head off, I finally realized that I'll never, ever be the same again. Not size, not shape, nor appearance. I stopped bawling, thinking, Well, if that's the case, then why am I trying to duplicate it? Why not become a new me? It doesn't make my 34B wrong. I loved that size. But, what if I welcome my newness without making the new size and shape wrong? It's just a new me. At that moment I decided to think of my new, literally "man-made" (never "fake") breasts as my "trophies!" That was my last meltdown for reconstruction.

§

The next day I saw my counselor and shared my new thought process. I was in a really good place—but now worried about the reaction I'd get when I'd requested "another fill" on the side I said was "way too big!" two weeks prior. Why on earth do we give others such power? I did ask for another fill; no comment was made other than, "Okay."

§

The neuropathy in my feet gradually faded. I could feel the inside of my shoes again. Just in time for a shoe sale! I decided to act on my good fortune. I tried on a pair of faux snakeskin boots. Three ladies I didn't know said, "O-ooo, you have to get those! They look so good on you!" (I never knew shoes could look good on someone! I mean, a top or a coat, yes—but shoes?) I got them. Hey, they were 65% off—and had a low heel!

§

Getting on the floor to stretch (no, not in my new boots!) I lost my balance. I've learned losing one's balance is common after a mastectomy. My hands were about five-inches from the floor. All my weight ended up on my right hand—without the strength to hold up my body. A week later my wrist still hurt, so I called the local health clinic. There was concern of brittle bones after chemo, but they believed this to be a sprain even though there'd been no swelling. They took X-rays. I left with a brace for what was thought to be a sprained wrist, and "trigger thumb." (When the tendon

Chapter 26

becomes inflamed and swollen, the finger and/or thumb catches or locks and isn't able to move freely. When it finally does move, the thumb will "pop", or "trigger" open, which is painful.)

I had physical therapy for my shoulders, balance, and posture gone awry. In addition to interim exercise homework, I swam at the pool a few times a week. Gradually I lost the ability to rotate my shoulders enough to get my arm out of the water no matter what stroke I'd do. So, I used a snorkel and mask, put my head down, and kick like crazy for thirty minutes—then go home and sleep for an hour or two.

§

April. I stopped going to the pool. My shoulders and "trigger thumb" hurt too much with the slightest wrong move. Five weeks after losing my balance, my wrist and thumb still hurt. I saw an orthopedist who made a cast to immobilize my thumb. I could remove the cast and often did. It put pressure on the very tendon needing relief. My hand puffed up a few times. I immediately removed the cast when I noticed swelling and did lymphedema exercises raising my arm high, opening and closing my hand. I ended up throwing out the cast.

Oncologists specialize in cancer treatment. If you need to go to a doctor who isn't part of a cancer treatment team, chances are very high that you know more about cancer than they do. Do not be shy to say no if you think there's a better way, or better doctor. I was used to my cancer clinic where everyone specializes in treating cancer. Then, I'd go to the emergency room, hospital, or other doctor and learn many, not all, are clueless about post-cancer needs. You must be your own advocate.

§

I heard from John. I knew things would move intensely fast when he returned. The direction in which they moved was bizarre. Surreal. Before he left, he'd confided in me he was looking for a new life, one that included marriage. Everything pointed to our being together. During the last 15 months while he'd been in Afghanistan, his three preteen kids made contact with their mother, living in another state. (They hadn't had contact in eight years.) Their mother began visiting them. Things moved along so well, mother and children began planning how family life would work when John came back to the USA. He was unaware of what was going on, not having access to communication. I guess they were all pretty convincing. He let me know he was remarrying the mother of his children after eight years of divorce, "So we can all move together overseas for my next assignment."

Wow. Ouch.

After hearing from John, I walked the beach with purpose, and repeated aloud the affirmation, "I accept my good." My prayers for "John or someone better" (which I believed to be John) had been answered loud and clear. This was the beginning of a long process in reminding myself, good doesn't always unfold in the ways we plan. I worked to change my perception on the outcome, trying to see it as good.

I'd walked an hour. The longest I'd walked in a year. I collapsed onto a mound of sand, knees first, then stiffly rolling over to sit. Immediately upon settling into the sand, I broke into sobs. Watching the shoreline, I thanked the retreating waves for taking my sorrow—while I wiped my tears in windshield wiper rhythm: right-left, right-left.

I said, "God, I'm really hurting. I need a spectacular gift today. Either outrageously funny, or stunningly beautiful. Bring it to me today, starting now." I was just about to stand up—a process that

Chapter 26

took time, and wasn't graceful with joint pain and limited range of motion.

Whoah! There must have been seventy-five dolphins in single file, passing up-close, right in front of me! I laughed, "Thanks God. That's a good one!" I watched them until they'd all passed. Dolphin totem stands for so much, but mostly a reminder to play and breathe, especially to release intense emotions. Dolphins tell us to move with the ebb and flow of life, and not to spend our energy fighting the current that gets us nowhere. Hmm . . . .

I slowly began to accept that my relationship with John moved from special to holy. I saw the gift was in the hope. Unknown to him, he was the carrot in front of me during my cancer treatment. Much of my getting stronger revolved around the vision I held of us together.

E-mail Updates
To: Bcc
Date: April 20

> *In June, I'll exchange the expanders for implants.*
>
> *Bye-bye to the port, which served me well, but I thank God I no longer need it.*

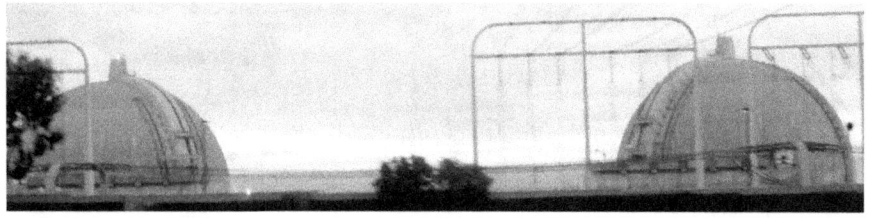

> *My implants will last about 12 years. It was explained to me like this: "It's like going to Costco for car tires. It's not fun, it takes up the entire day, it costs money, but it*

saves a blow out. It's something you just do." It's all so sexy, isn't it?

Very happy I've taken this slowly: Postponing the expansion start date a month to lessen the pain, and minimizing the amount of saline at each "fill up." I'm happy with the size I am now, which is a flip to where I was three months ago. I'm even okay with my hair at this stage.

Thanks all for your support. This comes one year and a day after I began chemo (6/3). Many people have told me I'm the first person they've known to live through chemo. Glad to hold that flag!

Health and Happiness,

Claudia

§

You are identifying with San Onofre? You see your new breasts as power plants or implants to power? You're obviously renewing your energy source and feeling more powerful.

You have made great progress and you are getting ready to cross the finish line to victory . . . .

Karen

§

Blessings of Love and Celebration for the progress you are making!

Namaste,

Rev John & Connie

Chapter 26

§

Dear Michelin,

You've carried the flag on so many levels for so many people.

cd

§

You look great by the way, even better than ever.

I'm good and hope you are as good as you look in your photo.

Be in touch again soon.

Cheers,

Allan

§

May. With my implant and port removal surgeries around the corner, I mopped the kitchen and bathroom floor for the first time since starting chemo a year ago. What a heartache. I realized how weak I'd become. I couldn't even squeeze the metal piece of the mop against the sponge to wring it out. I ended up using my leg to brace against the metal handle, and settled for a soggy sponge. End result: Sopping-wet but clean floor and incredible pain everywhere in my body.

The hideous shoulder pain I'd been experiencing for seven months was an impingement of the muscle that goes into the tendon at the rotator cuff. I continued with my physical therapy homework every other day. No lifting weights or doing anything causing pain or soreness. This was a really s-l-o-w process! I'd wake myself, moaning in pain. I couldn't take any pain relievers until after surgery.

June. Three hundred and sixty-six days after I began chemo, I claim my trophies, and relinquish my port!

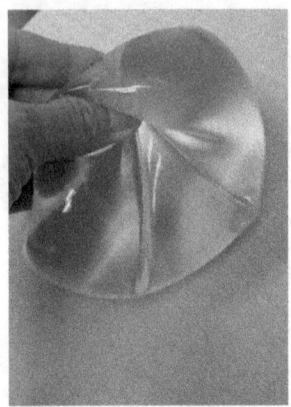

Silicone implants

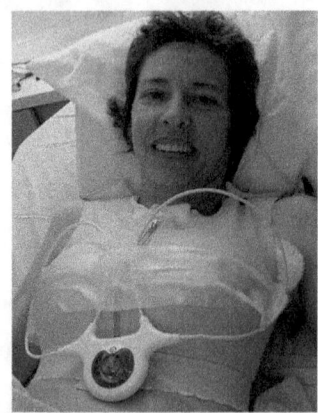

Recovery room; Ivivi SofPulse

I'd lined up help at home for the first week after surgery. I was more excited about this surgery than nervous—until a few days before. I don't know what happened, but I began freaking out. The day of surgery at the hospital I asked for a chaplain. "You need to request one." Uh . . . That's what I'm doing. They said, "You need to make an appointment for a chaplain to be at the hospital." The anesthesiologist arrived and told me to start thinking of pleasant things, and places. I'm usually really good at this. I couldn't think of a place—real or otherwise. I couldn't envision a calming or thrilling environment. Analytically, I knew God was in control. I knew I was safe. Other than that, I experienced far more fear going into this surgery than I did going into the bilateral mastectomy. I feared the outcome. I had approved this twelve to fifteen year implant commitment.

Three days after surgery I could open the after-surgery bra and look at the results. Pandora's Box. I unwrapped tons of padding

Chapter 26

and layers of gauze. When I got to the skin, I was both happy and horrified. For the expertise of artisan and skill of my surgeon I would forever be grateful. The size sent me into depression.

At my post-op appointment, the physician's assistant said, "Everything looks perfect." I spiraled further into panic about placement—which seemed off center on the right side—and size. I decided to wait and share my concerns with the surgeon at my next visit.

§

A year ago I thought I'd be celebrating at the port's removal. Instead, I was freaking out over the size of my new breasts. To me, they were huge! Clearing surgery papers from my kitchen counter I noticed: "375 cc." I flipped! On March 1, still with the half expanders, I had said, "This is the size I want" (240 cc). At that point, the surgeon only looked at projection, not shape. I understood the top portion wasn't filled, but also remembered the surgeon saying, "Perfect. You'll be a little smaller than that."

I spent the greater part of the week after surgery crying and depressed, and for two nights I sobbed like I did when first diagnosed. I bawled for hours, soaking my sheets. I didn't care if anyone heard. How the hell could this be so hard? The medical assistant kept telling me during the expander stage, "Most women give a general idea of the size they want, and aren't obsessed with the outcome. Most women say they wish they'd gone larger."

I've never fit into the "most women" category.

§

For the week after surgery I wore an Ivivi SofPulse. It's a bizarre looking apparatus that sends an electromagnetic pulse to lessen swelling, which decreases pain, which decreases the need for pain medication. Every few hours, this alien blinked green, calling its Mother Ship.

It worked, but they need to come up with a better system for securing it. It's taped on while the patient is lying in the hospital bed. The pretty satin ribbon-tape works great until the patient stands up. I tried four different types of tape. (Even duct tape didn't work and left ugly, sticky marks on the after-surgery bra.) The tapes all required tiresome adjustments throughout the day and none held the weight of the Ivivi SofPulse. I called the company. They suggested wearing SofPulse under the snug after-surgery bra. Yeah, right. Just try to fit it under the bra, and on top of freshly operated skin.

I'd been concerned how I'd get out of bed by myself after breast surgery, and now impinged rotator cuffs. Two days after surgery I was able to release my 24/7 help.

§

A few days after the "unveiling of my trophies," I realized I was slipping into depression again—something I hadn't been prone to before cancer. I'd hoped this surgery to be the start of one big happy dance. Mary picked me up and took me to her place, twelve miles inland. On the coast, the sun hadn't been out in a week. We both thought some sunshine would help me. We arrived at her house—met by a light summer rain. Inside, I took off my jacket then said, "I have to take a nap." I chose the brightest room and fell into a deep sleep for two and a half hours. When I awoke, we ate the dinner Mary made while I slept, then she shuttled me home. T'was a relaxing afternoon at Mary's daycare!

It took me ten days after surgery to come off the ledge of hysteria of my new breast size. It was time move to forward.

Chapter 26

§

The strangest thing about the implants: They're like molds of Jell-O, without the Midwestern whipped cream and marshmallows. Sometimes they're shockingly cold. Straight out of the refrigerator cold—which is a gross feeling when an arm skims the side of an implant while pulling off a shirt. The cold blob remains an element of surprise to me.

I've been given post-implant daily exercises to do for life. It's nothing earth shattering, but one more thing to do. Over time, I've grown to like these exercises. The implants feel less heavy and less cold after doing them. Basically, it's just squeezing the implants up, down and midline ten times. My oncology nurse mentioned, "You may hear a farting sound at high altitudes. They won't pop. Just talk loudly over the noise." Great.

§

The neurologist and I decided to increase my medication for neuropathy. "This increase is most likely temporary, but recovery may take one to two years. The nerves in your toes are farthest from the nerves in your spine, especially because you're tall." Neurontin made the difference between a slight buzz in my feet, or none at all.

My counselor completed her psychology doctoral internship at the cancer clinic. We had met a year prior, when things were really dark in my life. She wanted to work with children, so I promised to act more like one so she'd stay. She said, "You've been a bit of a challenge because you know of a lot of this stuff, but I've enjoyed working with someone who's aware of subtleties, and in tune with herself."

She was a safe person to witness my implosions. I could be me. Not the me I wanted to be, but the me I was in that very moment each week.

I'd share what was going on. She'd ask me, "How does that feel?"

I'd tell her what I thought. Projecting. Forecasting. At times reminiscing.

She'd return to my feelings. "Describe it."

I'd tell her my intentions, or fears.

She'd invite me to visit a certain feeling, asking, "What does that bring up for you?"

I fought it, not wanting to go negative. She pointed out my analytical answers to her questions about my feelings.

"OK, I'll play the game. Let's go." I journeyed to—and through—a very dark place with someone who'd hold the flashlight in one hand, and my hand in her other, bringing me to the darkness to shine the light.

§

July. The three apartments around me are vacant again! The obtuse neighbors who moved in with cancer left with it, too.

§

For the next year, lipstick was my only makeup. I couldn't be bothered using my energy applying anything more. I was a year into my chemo-induced menopause. To my absolute surprise it was b-a-a-a-ck. I couldn't believe it—nor was I celebrating the return of my menses. Ugh. (The last hurrah came again two weeks later, more like an exclamation point than a period.)

Chapter 26

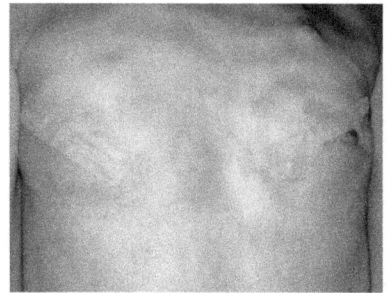

October: Two weeks after mastectomy

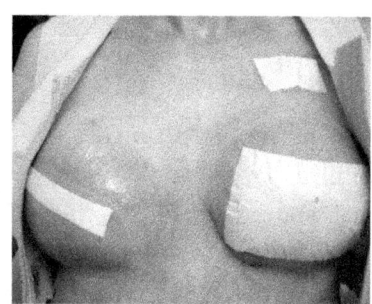

June: First implants Port removed

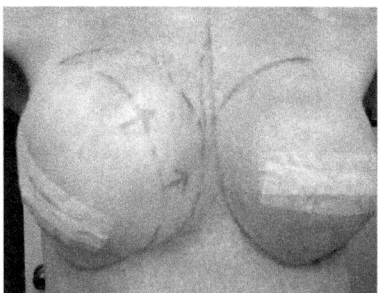

September: After third revision

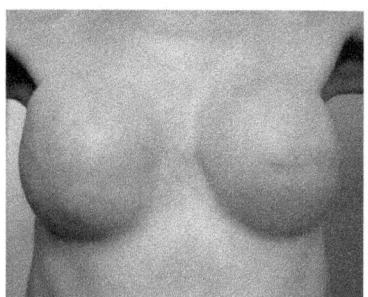

May: End result. A smaller, better fit for my frame and far more comfortable

§

September. I met a friend's relative who immediately after introduction asked, "Did you discover your breast cancer? Or was it through a test—or doctor visit?" I was blown away by this question! We hadn't established any rapport. I didn't mention cancer, nor was it part of our introduction.

I responded, "I'm not comfortable sharing that with you."
She replied, "I'm a nurse practitioner."
"Not mine."

§

The whole nipple thing was stressful. Should I get one? What were my options of how it would be done? Should I offer the one they spared back to the Nipple god? The spared nipple was permanently erect. It was very noticeable on my thin body. I wanted to walk down the street without poking anyone's eyes out.

Chapter 26

Tips for Him or Her:

✔ Bring a picture to the reconstruction surgeon if you have a certain image or size in mind.

✔ If you feel you aren't getting information, bring someone with you—maybe they can better communicate with your surgeon.

✔ Be willing to have a big, messy straight-talk appointment. You may not hear what you want, but you may hear some needed information you've missed along the way.

✔ Don't let anyone throw you off. People will share opinions and information that are none of their business. Some will question your vanity for having reconstruction. "Just wear a big shirt." Or, they'll tell you how they would cope if they had cancer. "If it were me, it'd be no big deal. I'm not vain." I felt I was entitled to reconstruction. Females have shape. It was my way of bringing me back to "whole"; my way of "filling the missing parts." I didn't want a daily reminder every morning and evening for the rest of my life while I arranged a prosthetic in a bra or swimsuit. Do what's right for you.

✔ Replace your pillows, wash your blankets, mattress pad, and anything else that may have stagnant energy. Flip your mattress. (I did this on my own and slept the greater portion of the day for doing so.) One day, I noticed my three-year-old couch had a seam ripping open. I called the store to see about having the rip repaired. They said, "That couch has a five year warranty. We'll swap it out." Talk about a fresh start!

Tips for Those Who Want to Help:

✔ Mind your P's and Q's. For those who like to ask questions, or who feel it's their job to share stories: If you haven't personally been through the procedures, consider keeping your mouth shut. This stuff can be horrifying to hear if it's going to happen to you—

especially if heard from someone who's never gone through any of it, but shares information as if it's common knowledge.

Chapter 27

TASSEL TWIRLING LESSONS POSTPONED

A revision surgery of June's reconstruction moved my right implant more median. This repositioned the implant that had gradually pulled itself toward the axilla.

At my post-operation appointment, I was told to wear a "push-up" bra round-the-clock for thirty days. "Make sure it really pushes you up, and in." I was told time and again that 32D was an "odd size." It took five stores to find a bra that fit. If they were "push-up," they were underwire, creating unbelievable pain. I got a bra, but it didn't nudge the right breast over as needed.

Another month passed. I had an appointment to talk about the nipple surgery. They would split the one I had on the left to make one on the right. "Someone will call you to schedule the surgery date."

Instead, two weeks later I called the surgeon asking him to look again at my situation. "My right breast hurts, especially midline. The discomfort dissipates when I hold my breast—something I try not to run around doing. The breast looks and feels like it's retreating toward my underarm."

The surgeon had me come in. "Indeed. The scar tissue has built-up and blocked the implant from naturally falling median." He postponed my nipple surgery and wrote me a six-week prescription for ultrasound, for the purpose of breaking up scar tissue. "If this doesn't break up the tissue, we'll need to create another pocket in which the implant will rest."

So much for getting a jump-start on those tassel twirling lessons this spring. Instead, I headed off to ultrasound. My right breast had moved back to almost where it was in January—before the revision.

§

Ultrasound didn't work. The physician's assistant said, "Schedule an appointment for surgery. He's pretty booked, but tell him you want a revision."

I waited two months for an appointment opening to talk about scheduling a revision of a previous revision—moving my right implant more median one more time. This pushed back my long awaited nipple several months. And, about six months after that, I'd have the opportunity to get my first tattoos (areolae), if I chose. Lydia, oh Lydia! It all came to a screeching halt.

§

A genetic counseling physician from the cancer clinic called me. "Your oncologist would like you to meet with me." The genetic counselor wanted to gather some family history to determine if I carried a high-risk ovarian cancer gene: BRCA I or II. "Knowing if you are a carrier could be a life saver to your younger female relatives."

"I'll meet with you, but I'm not sure how relevant this is for me."

During our one-hour session, she asked family history. "I don't have children. I have six nephews—no nieces. One aunt—she didn't have children. One uncle—he had one daughter, and five sons (one died of Hodgkin's). My mom's mother died at age forty-five; my dad's mother died at age twenty-six. That's all I know."

Chapter 27

My relatively young age at breast cancer diagnosis wasn't reason enough for a blood test. The lack of female history in my family raised the question: What would have happened had my grandmothers had lived longer?

"There's too much gray area to leave this alone. The good news for you—your odds of carrying the gene are lessened by not being Ashkenazi Jewish, or African American. In fact, Swedes and Italians (my ethnic backgrounds) have low BRCA gene rates. I'd like you to have the test anyway."

I agreed to the test, and waited a month for results (actually forgetting about them). I came home from a week at my mom's and had two messages from the genetic counseling department. Wow. They're good at follow-through. It was almost 5 p.m.; I figured I'd return their call before they left work. The doctor with whom I met a month ago answered the phone. She was pleasant, and good at what she did. Part of that was telling people, "I wish I had better news for you." I stood frozen. Grocery bags, and luggage at my feet. Unopened mail on the counter.

"What?!"

She continued, "Your test came back positive. I was shocked—"

I interrupted, babbling, and fully aware of it. "You're joking—April Fool's, right?—a day early?"

"No. I—"

Interrupting again, "—Of course, I know it's not a joke. It would be a bad one, anyway." Then I felt silly for rambling. I stopped and listened to her.

"There isn't much female history in your family, so it is a good thing you had the test."

I moved to the couch, now holding my head, tears flowing. "I know I'm going down the same road I did two years ago, but . . . could there be a mistake?"

"No. They tested two ways. Both came back positive. I'd like to schedule you to come in and we'll talk more in-depth about the next step. This will give you some time to absorb the shock before we move forward. It's not an emergency—but soon, having an oophorectomy—your ovaries removed—is in your best interest. Without that, you're a walking time bomb. The screening for ovarian cancer isn't good, and unlike breast cancer, the odds of survival with ovarian cancer are poor."

Oophowrectawho? They want to take my ovaries. From the appointment I had with her a month ago, I knew this was a possibility. But I was just going through the motions—it wasn't meant for me. I remained on the couch. Stunned. Numb. Opposing rationale ping-ponged in my head: I'm past childbearing age. They said taking ovaries perimenopausal or postmenopausal doesn't adversely affect the woman. From a month ago, I remembered her saying, "The ovaries are in retirement. If we need to, we take them out and send them on vacation." Sort of like a horse and glue.

Then my mind would bounce to the other side: It's not cancer. It's a preventive measure. Wow. Pretty drastic. The Body Snatchers. They see this as taking care of my body. This is my reasoning for why I took so long to go to the doctor two years ago.

Chapter 28

I KNOW THERE'S A PONY IN THIS PILE!

After a year and a half, my energy began to return. I began hiking, and doing sit-ups and push-ups again. My first push-up was more of a "push-down." I crashed into the carpet, making several attempts to push up.

My hair gradually thickened, and I remained hopeful that my hats would fit again. It was usually a near-balding man who'd say he didn't notice my hair was thin. Perhaps it was a polite way of saying, "Get over it."

At the time of writing, neuropathy is nearly gone, and my shoulder mobility is completely back. I still work on balance, and posture.

What I learned from cancer:

As a metaphysician, I'm always looking at "cause" in my life. Some people and books will offer a metaphysical view, and it's up to us to sit with that information to see if it fits for us—not to judge if it fits for anyone else. I didn't find a metaphysical "diagnosis" to fit for why I had cancer.

I believe before our souls enter our bodies, we help with the blueprint of our human experience. I get a mini video in my mind, and laugh when it plays. There I am, standing at the table with the chart of opportunities and choices laid out before me. I see myself making choices, and giving input, "Oh, I'll take the experience of cancer—but put it after I get my ministerial license. That way I'll know I'm a spiritual being having a human experience (not a human being having a spiritual experience), and I'll go through it easily." Ah, the eager soul!

Whatever the case, I had cancer. It wasn't easy, but it was made easier by my attitude of gratitude, and expectation to move through it with grace. Every single person who helped me (including strangers who smiled at me) blessed me, and were a part of my healing. No matter where you are on this journey, what type of cancer, or how many times you've walked this path, know you are whole, perfect, and complete.

Again,
I wish you peace. Deep Peace.
I wish you health, and happiness.
Blessings to you, and to those who help you.

Claudia

EPILOGUE

I wrestled whether I would include this portion in the book or not. My intention for this book was to uplift, not to scare.

I'd gone from "Stage 3, active cancer" to "Stage 2, non-active." Aware it could come back—believing it wouldn't. Believing plenty of people live long lives with non-active cancer (remission). I turned my back on further surgery, medication, and radiation. I was done.

Two years and two days after my first appointment with my surgical oncologist (the surgeon I'd seen for a second opinion, who removed the cancer), I had my last follow-up appointment with her. Immediately upon exam she said, "I see lymph nodes near your clavicle."

Déjà vu. Down the hallway for an ultrasound. The doctor preforming the ultrasound said, "Personally, I'm not comfortable taking a biopsy because the lymph nodes in question are near your jugular vein."

So, back down the hallway to the surgical oncologist. "I can do surgery next week." We heard a voice coming from the hallway. "—Wait . . . ." She stepped out of the room, then came back. Just my luck (really!): An ear, nose, and throat surgeon in the hallway just had a patient cancel. "Grab your things. He'll do your biopsy right now." I felt like the one-eyed, three-legged, deaf dog called "Lucky."

§

A nurse escorted me to a different room. I signed all sorts of consent forms. A minimum of four staff popped in the room, seemingly just to say, "This doctor's the best!" He entered the room. We had brief pleasantries. Soon I lay on the chair, now fully reclined, with my head downward.

The mood felt rather serious. "Umm . . . I have a job interview in two hours."

"You should be fine." He approached me with a long needle from the left, then the right. "I'm trying to figure which hand to use."

"Which is your dominant?"

Laughing, he said, "I'm pretty good with both."

I left with a Band-Aid and drove off to my interview. I got the job: Two hours a week for one month. It was a start to normalcy.

§

The following day, I got a call from the surgeon. I was re-diagnosed. This time my case was "unique and complicated." "Stage 4." (Later changing to "curable Stage 4.") The following week I began taking Tamoxifen, the medication I said I wouldn't take. Again my oncologist encouraged radiation. Again, I said, "No." This familiar discussion wrapped up with what seemed half-dare, half humor-me on the part of my oncologist: "Just hear the radiology oncologist out."

I agreed to a PET scan and consultation. For an hour and a half in the radiologist's office, I wailed. "You say this'll save my life, but I haven't regained one since chemo!" I donkey-legged on everything. "Tattoos and radiation—Auschwitz."

The radiology oncologist listened, but he didn't back down. For every push I gave, he pushed back. His voice was easy to listen to. He was firm without being harsh. "You say you're okay with death now, but you'll have four years—and they'll be painful at the end." With each bit of information, my head reeled. "Radiation is six-and-a-half weeks, Monday through Friday." He handed me the box of thin, scratchy hospital tissues. (I still showed up to doctor appointments thinking I wouldn't need to bring my own.) Drilling him with question after question, I left without a follow-up appointment. I couldn't guarantee I'd be back.

Four months later, I returned. I told the doctor he was the main reason. "I appreciate how you worked with me. You were honest, respectful, and not a pushover."

He smiled and said, "So I did my job?"

§

After three months on Tamoxifen, a new tumor could be felt. The day after my ovaries were removed, my medication was switched to Femara. A month later, the tumors stopped growing, but remained two centimeters in size. They needed to be less than one centimeter for me to receive a smaller amount, and streamline delivery of radiation. We were running out of options. The doctors began considering I.V. chemo again. The third medication worked. For me, Aromasin made Tamoxifen's side effects seem like candy—but the tumors shrunk.

§

Radiation was psychologically harder for me than chemo or surgery—but easier on my body. Waiting eight months for tumors to shrink before beginning radiation may have added to the stress and feeling of impending doom. I clung to every word of encouragement from my radiology oncologist. He received more pushback from me than any other on my medical team. One month before radiation, a small dot was tattooed on my chest, and each axilla to ensure exact positioning for six weeks of radiation treatment. Being tattooed was very close to a deal breaker for me. I began another "Wall of Gratitude." Two weeks into radiation, something shifted. All the spiritual, mental, and emotional work I'd done finally shattered my resistance. It happened while I was driving. All of a sudden it felt like a glass vase tightly surrounded me—then broke. I felt light—not euphoric, but the heaviness and dread lifted. I knew I'd be okay. From that night on, I could lie on my bed and not associate it with being on the radiation table. (The sensation of the radiation table locking into place transferred to my bed, and kept me up every night prior.)

§

Less than two months after completing radiation, I had the tattoos removed. I told the guy at the tattoo shop, "These will be the smallest and most important tattoos you'll ever remove." Then I did my show and tell.

His eyes opened wide, "I knew you looked familiar! You came to the hospital to take a picture of the port catheter for your book, and you brought me lunch because I told you on the phone I wasn't taking a lunch that day." He worked at the hospital during the week. On Saturdays he removed tattoos.

Zap. Zap. Zap. It was done. I immediately felt whole and on top of the world! In many cases, it's highly recommended—sometimes insisted—that tattoos stay.

§

Unlike some, I got to hear, "You are cancer free" (Stage 4, no evidence of disease). My immediate reaction was to complain—even cry for still having neuropathy, subclinical lymphedema, and flat, thin hair. Then, things began shifting. I saw my energy coming back, and six months later, the revision of a revision that had been postponed due to re-diagnosis happened. Finally! Three years and

Epilogue

six surgeries later. I asked that my spared nipple—something I was so grateful for—be removed rather than having a seventh surgery to split and create a new nipple. Giving up a nipple. Is this what they mean by tit for tat? (Who is Tat, anyway?) I also decided to forego tattooed areolae. If Barbie can make it without nipples and areolae, so can I!

§

Six months later I had a third revision, bringing me to the seventh surgery I'd aimed to avoid. The new style of implants used in the previous surgery were so heavy, they brought my posture to a forward slant. The size was even bigger than the original implants that sent me into such a tailspin. The style was "teardrop," which made my figure look frumpy and in need of a lift, and one side was puckering. The rough texture of the new implants was intended to hold them in place by grabbing muscle in my chest wall. The muscle was grabbed all right. I was in constant pain. I began to breathe shallow breaths to avoid pain. One day my mom gave me a hug and she repelled back in shock. We'd both been physically hurt by the hug as if I'd had two bricks in shirt pockets.

Enough!

I found a new surgeon who won points with me when she asked, "Are you happy with this shape and size?" I grabbed my notebook and all the reasons to eventually answer, "No." She eyed my body, "It's a bit large for your frame." I downsized from 370 cc to 325 cc. This revision surgery was the least painful of the three.

Now, my posture is great again. I recognize and like who I see in the mirror, and I am comfortable.

§

Two years and three months later: Third time's a charm? One evening, I ran my hands down my neck and across my shoulders. I felt a bump on my back, between my neck and shoulder. Uh-oh. The self-talk began. Of course. It's a pulled muscle from sanding my bookcase a few days ago. I felt the bump again. No way! It felt just like the ones four years ago in my armpit, and two years ago in the front of my neck.

I'm considered "high risk", and am supposed to call my oncologist if I ever have questions, or a suspicious bump. After an hour of asking for inner-guidance, and twisting around to look in the mirror to see it with my own eyes, I made the phone call to leave a message. It was Friday night. "Hi! I'm calling because I'm supposed to. I just noticed a tiny bump. It's the size of a mosquito bite—pretty small. I think it's a pulled muscle. I'm going out of town Tuesday to see my dad. I've got an appointment scheduled to come in when I return in two weeks."

I got a return call Monday morning. "Come in tomorrow morning."

"I'm leaving tomorrow night. I don't have time to drive back and forth to the clinic, to turn around and head to the airport."

"Come in 2 p.m. Tuesday."

Bags packed, I headed out to my oncologist. He felt the bump. "When do you leave?"

"Right after this appointment."

"How long will you be gone?"

"Two weeks."

He walked the razor's edge of informing me, while trying not to push any buttons. "Keep your appointment that's already scheduled for when you get back. If I were to guess, I'd say it's cancer, but I don't want to guess. We'll get blood work and a biopsy when you return. Have a great time. Don't let this wreck your trip."

I added one thing, "You know, the two times I was diagnosed before this were each two years apart form each other. Both times, I was diagnosed the week of my mom's birthday. Here we are—two years out again. This week is my dad's birthday. How do you even tell a parent cancer's back for the third time?"

"It's just a guess. I have no proof yet, but I want you to be prepared."

I left the office. No tears, no swearing. I didn't tell my dad until the day before my flight home. I didn't tell my mom until a week after I returned from the trip. Telling my parents that cancer was back was the hardest thing I ever had to tell them. It took over a month to tell my best friends. Not one person from my e-mail update list knew until a month passed. This time, cancer had a very different feel. It was eerie.

When I did tell my friend, Mary, we were outside on a beautiful day. Immediately after I told her, "Cancer's back" we heard a hawk screech. We looked up. There was a red-tailed hawk circling above. Oh, what a sight! We took in the moment, sitting in silence. Here I was, four years later, again receiving a red-tailed hawk totem message: Pull back, broaden your focus. Keep the analytical mind under control, not allowing it to run wild. Where hard work is involved, so are great rewards . . . . What a gift. Then the hawk flew away.

§

I had a month of blood tests, more blood tests, scans, x-rays, and a biopsy needed to be redone. It came back negative, but I was getting more bumps, and they were getting larger. The medical team thought for sure it would come back positive. With previous cancer diagnosis, I'd had two biopsies come back negative, then after surgery, they were re-tested—and they came back positive. Hearing the results were negative was great, but I needed to completely believe it.

A bone density scan showed a drop in my bone density. A blood test showed elevated calcium levels. The two together meant the bones weren't absorbing the calcium. My doctor wanted to rule out bone cancer. I was asked if my tailbone hurt at all. It did hurt while picking up trash at the beach weekly, but I blew it off as being out of shape, and thought I needed to do more "beach beautification workouts." I had x-rays after the bone scan because they saw the radioactive dye collect at my sacrum. The nurse practitioner said, "It's either a hairline fracture, or cancer. Stop activities that aggravate it." The x-rays were to show a better view of my tailbone. Next, CT Scan, and a bone biopsy. I was told it would feel like I'd been kicked in the tailbone a few days after the sacrum biopsy. Unfortunately, that was a very good analogy.

Treatment for metastatic breast cancer began. This time, I only had ten days of radiation because my spine was being radiated. I was ready, and able to hold my head high. I did ask for—and got tape radiation markers rather than tattoos. My radiology oncologist was comfortable with the tape markers for only ten days and knowing I was determined to keep the markers in place.

The radiation team commented on how calm I was everyday. I laughed and told them to let my prior team know. At graduation, I rang that same bell I had the year prior. One ring. One loud, clear ring. When I got home I noticed my radiation end-date for this round was the same month and day as my previous radiation start-date.

§

The first time, I didn't say "no" to radiation because of fear alone. It took major soul-searching. I prayed, meditated, and felt guided to say "no" at the time. I truly felt removing more lymph nodes, taking Tamoxifen, and undergoing radiation weren't in my best interest. The second time I still said, "no"—then did more soul-searching. Unknown to us, sometimes "no" means "not now." The surgery to remove more lymph nodes was not suggested the second time with my moving forward with medication and radiation.

I look back on this process with gratitude for my listening to guidance. If I'd taken Tamoxifen for two years, I might have still had tumor growth. By my saying "no" to radiation two years earlier, I was a clean slate for this round. (They can't radiate the same area twice.) Declining surgery also worked in my favor, as they decided I could take a pass.

Please don't read this as my promoting you not following your treatment plan. But do remember you are a member on your treatment team. Listen to them, and follow your guidance. When you're in fear, you'll hear the ego; the small-self; the analytical mind. That's not guidance. Trust your medical team. Trust yourself. Trust that place you turn to for guidance.

§

I hope your cancer experience is like a diamond, an earthquake, and learning to float. Claim your beauty and strength from the pressures and heat endured throughout this process. Rebuild your foundation once shaken by the earthquake. Trust. Float.

Epilogue

Tips for Him or Her:

✔ Find the ability to trust—whether it's in a higher power, your medical team, yourself, others, or all of these.

✔ Focus on what's working in your life. Where's the good? For whom and what are you grateful? Every day, throughout the day, find things for which to be grateful—even if it's only one—even if it's almost sarcastic. Has the pain or nausea stopped? Are your bills paid? Sheets clean? Do you have a spot of beauty at which to look? Did you hear the birds sing today? Are you glad you're alive? (And if not, find something to focus on that shifts the darkness to light.)

✔ Before chemo, I found the word "Smile" in a magazine. I taped this five-inch reminder on my vanity mirror. There is reason to smile during all this. Find at least one reason everyday. A few other affirmations already on my mirror from years past: "Go confidently in the direction of your dreams"—Henry David Thoreau. "I unconditionally love myself," and, "I boldly believe the Universe is working this out in an amazing, quick and perfect way. A way that leaves me filled with joy and gratitude!"

✔ Ask yourself, "What will I do today to make myself happy?" It's along the same lines of committing to "fall in love three times a day." Fall in love with the sound of a bird chirping, the sight of a flower blooming, the feel of a gentle hand on your shoulder. Fall in love with the expression of life. Look around!

✔ Let the airline know if you're flying to receive medical treatment. If you need to change your flight date, the airlines will often keep your ticket price the same, even if the ticket fare is more for the newer date.

RESOURCES

American Cancer Society (ACS):
1-800-ACS-2345 (1-800-227-2345), www.cancer.org
Offers a variety of services to patients and their families.

Breast Cancer:
www.breastcancer.org
Committed to providing complete, accurate, and private cancer information.

CancerCare:
1-800-994-HOPE (1-800-994-4673), www.cancercare.org
Counseling. Support Groups. Education. Financial Assistance.

Certified Hypnotherapist, Brennan P. Smith, C.Ht:
www.BrennanSmith.com
Therapeutic Hypnosis cds and mp3s.

Charity Navigator:
www.charitynavigator.org
Research before donating to charity! Charity Navigator is an independent charity evaluator, providing information on over 5,000 charities.

Chronic Disease Fund:
www.cdfund.org
Assists patients through the United States with chronic disease, cancer and other life-altering conditions obtain the life-saving medications they need, and travel assistance.

Patients must meet income qualification guidelines and have private insurance or a Medicare Part D plan but cannot afford the cost of their specialty therapeutics.

Cleaning for a Reason:
www.cleaningforareason.org
Providing maid service for patients undergoing treatment for any type of cancer.

State Disability Insurance (SDI):
SDI is in *only five states* (CA, HI, NJ, NY, RI, and the Commonwealth of Puerto Rico)
CA: 1-800-480-3287, www.edd.ca.gov
HI: 808-586-9161, www.labor.hawaii.gov
NJ: 609-292-7060, www.nj.gov/labor
RI: 401-462-8420, www.dlt.ri.gov/tdi
Puerto Rico: 809-754-2119

Paid Family Leave (PFL):
PFL for caregivers is in only two states (CA, NJ)
CA: 1-877-238-4373, www.edd.ca.gov
NJ: 609-292-7060, www.nj.gov/labor

Lymphology Association of North America (LANA):
www.clt-lana.org
A list of Certified LANA Therapists.

Mederma:
www.mederma.com
Scar reduction product.

National Cancer Institute (NCI):
1-800-4-CANCER (1-800-422-6237), www.cancer.gov
NCI is part of the National Institutes of Health and the Department of Health and Human Services. NCI's main responsibilities include coordinating the National Cancer Program; conducting and supporting cancer research; training physicians and scientists; and

disseminating information about cancer detection, diagnosis, treatment, prevention, control, palliative care, and survivorship.

National Hospice and Palliative Care Organization (NHPCO):
1–800–658–8898, www.caringinfo.org
Free resources and information re: end-of-life care, and services before a crisis.
It's About How You LIVE - a campaign with community, state and national partners to improve end-of-life care.

NeedyMeds:
www.needymeds.org
NeedyMeds is not a patient assistance program. A source of free information on thousands of programs that may be able to offer medications and healthcare cost assistance to people in need. Free prescription discount card is active immediately and never expires. Anyone can use the card as there are no income, insurance, age, or residency requirements.

ScarLine Rx:
www.scarline.com
Scar reduction product.

Social Security (SS):
1-800-772-1213, www.socialsecurity.gov
Find your local office.

ABOUT THE AUTHOR

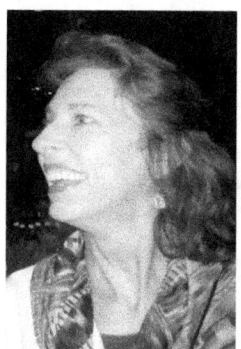

Claudia Mulcahy

Claudia's passion is teaching, demonstrating and inspiring people to live at higher levels of consciousness. She embraces universal spiritual new thought concepts, and holds a ministerial license with Emerson New Thought Center, Church Without Walls. Claudia is a native of San Diego, California. She lives her life in gratitude and loves to spend time in positive environments, nature and traveling. She also enjoys time spent with her parents, and other loved ones. Claudia is thriving, and living every day to the fullest. Visit Claudia at www.CancerWhatToDoOrSay.com.

www.ingramcontent.com/pod-product-compliance
Lightning Source LLC
Chambersburg PA
CBHW050626300426
44112CB00012B/1671